EMPOWERED AGAINST CANCER

SCIENCE-BASED STRATEGIES TO OPTIMIZE YOUR TREATMENTS AND THRIVE

A PRACTICAL GUIDE

BRIAN LAWENDA, M.D., CONNER MIDDELMANN

MW00658281

Author names: Brian Lawenda MD, Conner Middelmann

Edition: First edition

Year of publication: 2021

ISBNs:

Kindle: 978-1-7367935-1-0

Print: 978-1-7367935-0-3

Collaborators:

Editors: Elisa Boseley, Siobhan Gallagher

Cover artist: Jasmine Hromjak

Type setting: Codruţ Sebastian Făgăraş

Author photographs: James Cavanagh, Kirsten Boyer

All rights reserved. No part of this publication may be reproduced, stored or transmitted in any form or by any means, electronic, mechanical, photocopying, recording, scanning, or otherwise without written permission from the publisher. It is illegal to copy this book, post it to a website, or distribute it by any other means without permission.

Brian Lawenda, MD, and Conner Middelmann assert the moral right to be identified as the authors of this work.

Brian Lawenda, MD, and Conner Middelmann have no responsibility for the persistence or accuracy of URLs for external or third-party Internet Websites referred to in this publication and do not guarantee that any content on such Websites is, or will remain, accurate or appropriate.

Designations used by companies to distinguish their products are often claimed as trademarks. All brand names and product names used in this book and on its cover are trade names, service marks, trademarks and registered trademarks of their respective owners. The publishers and the book are not associated with any product or vendor mentioned in this book. None of the companies referenced within the book have endorsed the book.

This publication contains the opinions and ideas of its authors. It is intended to provide educational material on the subjects addressed in the publication. It is sold with the understanding that the authors are not engaged in rendering medical, health or any other kind of personal or professional services in the book. If the reader requires personal medical, health or other assistance or advice, a certified health professional should be consulted. Although every care and precaution has been taken in the preparation of this book, the authors specifically disclaim all responsibility for any liability, loss or risk, personal or otherwise, that is incurred as a consequence, directly or indirectly, of the use and application of any of the contents of this book. Before undertaking significant dietary or lifestyle changes, check with your doctor whether these changes are appropriate and safe for you.

To all the people we have had the privilege of supporting over the years. You have taught us deep lessons about courage, love and grace, and you inspire us to keep learning so we can better serve you and others.

Brian Lawenda, M.D., Conner Middelmann

CONTENTS

FOREWORD

by Donald I. Abrams, M.D., Professor Emeritus of Medicine, University of California San Francisco; Integrative Oncologist, UCSF Osher Center for Integrative Medicine

One of the primary goals of integrative oncology is to return to the individual a sense of control. When one hears the words "You have cancer," it is as if the rug has been pulled out from under you. You are now at the mercy of the surgeon, the radiation oncologist, the medical oncologist, and the chemotherapy nurse.

For many, this can be a very disturbing, even disorienting, experience. Consultation with an integrative care provider can help restore that sense of control.

I often tell patients I see in my integrative oncology consultation practice that cancer is like a weed: other people are taking care of their weed and it's my job to work with the garden and make their soil as inhospitable as possible to growth and spread of the weed. I do that by seeing how they fertilize the garden; that is, what they eat and what supplements they take.

We now appreciate that diet and weight likely contribute to more malignant diagnoses than tobacco use! By encouraging an organic, plant-based, antioxidant-rich, anti-inflammatory whole foods diet, I offer the patient the opportunity to regain a sense of having some control in their journey, as well as an alternative to the conventional oncologist's mantra to "Eat whatever you want; it doesn't really matter!"

The conventional cancer care provider might also be very emphatic in advising patients not to take any supplements during cancer treatment that they have not been prescribed. Clearly, they are concerned that something may interfere with their therapy, making it less effective or more toxic. But the integrative oncologist knows what supplements are most likely safe and hopefully will be beneficial for the patient to incorporate into their regimen. This also offers the individual further opportunity to be more directly involved in their prescription toward wellbeing.

Physical activity not only decreases the risk of cancer but has been shown to improve outcomes in breast, prostate, and colon cancer. Most patients would like their oncologist to recommend or advise them on an exercise regimen, but only a minority do so. Let's face it, trying to keep up with the treatment advances in each segment of cancer care is enough of a challenge. Expecting your oncologist to advise you on aerobic and resistance activities may be expecting too much. Yoga has been shown to improve quality of life in numerous clinical trials in cancer patients.

When I ask a new patient to "tell me your story," people often weave a narrative suggesting that stress may have caused their cancer. Although I do not think stress in and of itself can cause cancer, stress is not good for cancer—or for anything else, for that matter. Stress is epinephrine, which kills the lymphocytes, the building blocks of the immune system, and cortisol, a steroid hormone that is an immune suppressant. So decreasing stress is another goal of integrative cancer care, and we have many modalities to recommend to that end.

You are holding in your hands a veritable gold mine of integrative cancer care. Brian and Conner have gifted us with a comprehensive, comprehensible, and compassionate guidebook for navigating life after a cancer diagnosis. They cover all the bases: nutrition, supplements, physical activity, stress reduction, and spirituality. Their advice is sound, science-informed, and easy to digest. They offer sound recommendations and clearly outline next steps under the "Over to You" headings, facilitating the reader's ability to really make the suggested changes.

I ask everyone I see on our first visit three questions: *What brings you joy? What are your hopes? Where does your strength come from?* No matter where the individual is on the journey with cancer, I feel it is important to remember that they still do have joy, hope, and strength. Reading this empowering handbook (or guide) will certainly leave you with a healthy dose of all three. To your health!

PREFACE

by Brian Lawenda, M.D.
Radiation Oncologist and Integrative Oncologist
Founder, IntegrativeOncology-Essentials
and the IOEProgram

Every morning after I wake up, I drink my coffee and start reviewing the latest medical news and journal articles. This review process continues all day, every day: on breaks between patients, after work, weekends. Over the past 20 years, I conservatively estimate that I've spent more than 13,000 hours reading about the evolving science of cancer.

At the same time, as a radiation oncologist, integrative oncologist, medical acupuncturist, and functional medicine practitioner, I've logged more than 48,000 clinic hours managing the complex care of thousands of cancer patients. My co-author, Conner Middelmann, has likewise spent thousands of hours studying nutrition and counseling cancer patients on the specifics of how and what to eat.

For years, Conner and I have been working together on a book to help answer the most commonly asked questions we hear and to provide people with essential and actionable information they can use before, during, and after cancer treatments. Our initial book draft was over 350 pages long. *Oy vey!*

We quickly realized that no one would have the energy to read a long-winded book groaning with research references, statistics, tables, and charts. Instead, we decided to condense this heavily researched information into an easy-to-use handbook that can serve as a guide for people with cancer, and that every oncologist and cancer center library could recommend. (Research references are available upon request.)

If you were recently diagnosed with cancer, you'll have lots of questions. Searching the internet and getting advice from friends and family are usually the first places people turn, and you'll likely continue to use these tools.

But despite months to years of being in and out of an oncologist's clinic, many people never learn the information they need to help them get through treatments more easily or to create a customized lifestyle strategy to optimize their cancer outcome and quality of life.

We hope that instead of spending countless hours looking for answers that may or may not be trustworthy, you'll reach for this handbook to quickly learn the foundational strategies that you and all cancer patients and survivors need to know.

Brian Lawenda, M.D., April 2021

P.S. Throughout this guide we recommend products, services, and publications that we hope will be useful to you. We do not receive any financial benefit from these recommendations. Our only sources of revenue are from our clinical work, sales of my IOE program, and Conner's books and courses.

ACKNOWLEDGMENTS

BL: I want to acknowledge the following physicians, researchers, and mentors who have helped shape my knowledge of medicine and my practice and care of cancer patients and survivors: Donald Abrams, M.D., Keith Block, M.D., Paul Busse, M.D., Jeffrey Blumberg, M.D., Lorenzo Cohen, M.D., Thomas Delaney, M.D., Daniel Doseretz, M.D., David Eisenberg, M.D., Joseph Helms, M.D., Rakesh Jain, M.D., Peter Johnstone, M.D., Lisa Kachnic, M.D., Daniel Kalish, M.D., Jay Loeffler, M.D., Constantine Mantz, M.D., James McIntyre, M.D., Paul Mills, M.D., Simon Powell, M.D., Stephen Sagar, M.D., Herman Suit, M.D., Alphonse Taghian, M.D., Nancy Tarbell, M.D., Christopher Willett, M.D., and Anthony Zietman, M.D. I will be forever grateful for your friendships and guidance. I want to give a special acknowledgment to my wife, Jenni, my biggest supporter.

CM: Heartfelt thanks to my co-author Brian—not only for inviting me to collaborate on this book and for teaching me so much about integrative oncology but also for being an exceptionally kind and generous human being. During a prolonged, stressful transition in my personal life, Brian, with the patience of a saint, let me take the time I needed to tackle my challenges while continuing to work on this book at a much slower pace than either of us had anticipated. Another big thank-you to Elisa Bosley, our fearless editor, who managed to condense 350-odd pages of science-speak into a breezy read. Much gratitude, too, to Cari Dawson,

M.D., and Alex Goldsmith, M.D., at the Colorado Center of Medical Excellence, who have taught me so much; to Nanna Bo Christiansen at Boulder Community Health's cancer center for hosting my nutrition workshops; Jacob Schor, N.D., for enthusiastically sharing his encyclopedic knowledge of cancer and nutrition with me; and to the late David Servan-Schreiber, M.D., for introducing me to integrative oncology. Last, but not least, my deepest gratitude goes to all the wonderful people who cheered me on, cooked for me, provided support and wise counsel during tough times, lent me their cabin for writing retreats, and forgave me the many weekends spent at the computer: Stewart Walker, Vicky and John Graham, Bryan Handwork, Sukmi and Pascal Ledru, Hanna and Wolf Middelmann, Anke Middelmann, Will Menaker, Eva Szita-Morris, and my beloved children, Charlotte, Max, and Oscar.

Chapter 1

Really?
Another Book About Cancer?

"Keto for cancer." "Veganism for cancer." "Running for cancer." "Juicing for cancer." Yes, we know; there are already myriad self-help books for people with cancer. Some are excellent, some a little more dubious.

We're not here to reinvent the wheel or to propose a definitive cancer cure (spoiler alert: there isn't one). Rather, we want to empower you—and your doctor—to add easy, evidence-based complementary therapies to your standard treatments to improve your outcome and quality of life.

Change Is Happening

Depending on the region and state where you live, cancer is the No. 1 or 2 killer in America. But cancer is changing. Even as more people are diagnosed with the disease, more people are surviving. A cancer diagnosis is no longer a life-or-death sentence; instead, it's increasingly seen as a chronic disease that can be managed over years, and even decades.

How is this change happening? Standard cancer treatments (surgery, chemotherapy, radiation, hormone therapy, and more) are undoubtedly improving, but that's not all. Studies increasingly show that people who combine complementary therapies—including diet, exercise, meditation, and more—with conventional cancer treatments have better outcomes than those who don't.

I, Dr. Lawenda, am an oncologist, first and foremost. What makes me different from many cancer doctors is my belief that the cancer journey is more successful and leads to better quality of life when state-of-the-art cancer treatments are combined with evidence-based, holistic strategies that enhance your body and mind's natural anticancer abilities.

I, Conner Middelmann, am a nutritionist and 21-year cancer survivor. In 2007, I read *Anticancer: A New Way of Life* by David Servan-Schreiber, M.D., PhD, which inspired me to write a nutrition guide and cookbook, *Zest for Life: The Mediterranean Anti-Cancer Diet.* I now support people with cancer through in-person and online coaching, recipes and meal plans, webinars, and cooking classes.

Together, our goal is to show you, a person with cancer, practical ways to play an active role in your cancer treatment. We believe that considering and using every possible research-backed treatment will empower you in this journey—an attitude that in itself can profoundly impact your recovery.

Your Doctor, Your Partner

Most oncologists know a lot about treating cancer with standard therapies. But when was the last time a doctor sat you down for one, two, or three hours and taught you about all the things you could do to reduce your risks of cancer growth, spread, and recurrence?

You can't really blame the doctor. Most oncologists' clinic schedules are already maxed out. They don't get reimbursed for spending extra time to become trained in or to discuss topics that seem to fall outside the typical scope of cancer care.

Nearly one-third of people in the U.S. with cancer already use complementary treatments—often without the knowledge of their doctor. Cancer patients who keep quiet about complementary treatments may think that their medical providers aren't knowledgeable in these therapies, or worry that their doctors will be dismissive or upset with them and tell them to stop, even if the person with cancer feels the complementary therapies are helping.

Aside from the worrying lack of trust—and trust is crucial in any doctor–patient relationship—there can be downsides and even physical risks when people don't tell their healthcare providers about complementary therapies or lifestyle interventions. Alternative approaches, when not disclosed, may lead to dangerous interactions with medications, unintended and avoidable side effects, reduced treatment efficacy, delays in starting standard treatments, and more.

We don't want you to stop complementary therapies. But we encourage you to be honest with everyone on your care team. When done safely and with the knowledge of your entire oncology team, alternative approaches and lifestyle changes combined with standard treatments can improve your cancer outcome.

Fighting Cancer on All Fronts

We're sure you know someone—maybe a computer technician—who, when called to resolve your problem, launches into a highly technical monologue about what caused the problem, how he figured it out, and what he did to resolve it. As your eyes glaze over, you think: "All I wanted was for him to fix my laptop—not a degree in computer science." As an oncologist and nutritionist, we often see the same thing.

When you're in the middle of a crisis such as a new cancer diagnosis or a difficult treatment, you want solutions, not explanations. That's not to say the explanations aren't important. But there's a time for detailed explanations and a time for problem-solving. That's what this book is for.

We provide quick and easy strategies for people who've recently received a cancer diagnosis or who may be struggling with treatment side effects. We are not saying that acupuncture, dietary changes, or a daily walk will cure your cancer. What we are saying is that the evidence-informed complementary therapies we describe can give you an active, effective role in working to overcome cancer, help boost your anticancer defenses, improve the outcome of your treatments, lift your spirits, and enhance your enjoyment of life.

Creating the Right Environment

The idea of creating an environment in the body that's inhospitable to cancer isn't new. As long ago as 1889, British cancer doctor Stephen Paget noted, "Every single cancer cell must be regarded as an organism, alive and capable of development. When a plant goes to seed, its seeds are carried in all directions; but they can only live and grow if they fall on congenial soil."

In this book, we show how you can create a "soil" (tissue environment) in your body that makes cancer cells feel very unwelcome. Better still, studies show that the lifestyle measures we discuss can reduce the risk of your cancer coming back, once your treatment is complete.

We hope this book eventually finds its way onto every oncologist's desk, so that when faced with the difficult task of telling a person they have cancer, the doctor will be able to add this encouragement: "We'll do everything we can to help you beat cancer. And in addition to possible surgery, chemotherapy, and radiation, there are many things you can do to improve the outcome of your treatment. Here, take a copy of this handbook and learn what you can do to help us."

How to Use This Book

Like most how-to guides, this book isn't intended to be read from cover to cover. Each section contains short chapters on specific issues relevant to people with cancer. Each chapter includes action points for things you can do right away.

If you're newly diagnosed and preparing for treatment, start by flipping through the book or scanning the index to see what jumps out at you. If you're already undergoing treatment and have specific questions related to cancer, read the relevant chapter(s) and start implementing the recommendations.

Don't try to do everything at once. Not all interventions suit every person, and when you take on too much, you risk unnecessary stress and a loss of focus. It's better to do a few things well than several things haphazardly.

We recommend that you make changes gradually. For instance, start by eating an additional serving of vegetables each day. Once you're happily doing this, increase it to two. Next, try to go for a 20- to 30-minute walk every day. Once that's part of your daily routine, include a 10-minute meditation before breakfast. And so on. It takes most people at least one to two months (and often longer) before a new practice becomes an automatic habit, so keep at it.

People are more likely to stick with healthy behaviors if they enjoy them (or at least find them manageable). So, out of the many ideas in this book, start with those that feel easy and make you feel good. Any regularly practiced healthy behavior—no matter how modest—will support you on the road to surviving cancer.

Controlling the Controllables

Every living organism is a constant work in progress. Cells, the building blocks of life, grow, divide, and grow some more. The cells that line your intestine, for example, renew themselves roughly every three days, skin cells are replaced every 20 days, red blood cells every four months, and liver cells every six months.

At every step of this process, cell growth needs to be tightly controlled. If it isn't, every organism would keep growing indefinitely. Nature has many mechanisms that turn cell growth on and off.

Cancer develops when these controls fail. When there's nothing to stop cells from growing, cancer cells multiply in an unregulated manner.

Humans can influence some of these cancer triggers, but many are beyond our control. That's why it's important that you don't blame yourself for your cancer. While factors (such as exposure to cancer-causing agents) and choices (such as smoking) may have influenced your cancer risk, they didn't cause your cancer.

Now it's time to look at all the things you can influence: your diet, physical activity patterns, stress levels, sleep habits, and priorities. Taking charge of these areas can:

- Give your treatment the best chances of succeeding
- Speed your recovery from treatment
- Reduce the chances of the cancer coming back

With the help of a comprehensive anticancer lifestyle approach and other interventions, you can influence whether your body is hospitable vs. hostile to cancer cells.

What Is Integrative Oncology?

Integrative oncologists focus on the whole person as a complex system comprising mind, body, and spirit. Rather than only focusing on killing the cancer, an integrative practitioner examines the environment in which the cancer developed in the first place, and advises the patient on ways to support their body's own defenses against cancer, for instance by lowering inflammation or reducing stress levels to strengthen immunity.

Integrative oncology combines three essential components:

1. Conventional cancer treatments, such as chemotherapy, surgery, and radiation therapy
2. Lifestyle counseling, such as nutrition, exercise, stress reduction, smoking cessation, and toxin avoidance
3. Complementary therapies, such as botanical supplements, massage, acupuncture, and meditation

This three-pronged approach boosts the body's innate ability to fight and prevent cancer. In this way, integrative oncologists help to create an environment—or "terrain"—in the body that makes it harder for cancer cells to thrive.

Integrative oncology has another goal: to empower you to play an active role in your treatment. A cancer diagnosis sucks many intelligent, independent-minded people into a "cancer machine" that makes them feel as though they've lost all control over their life and become passive recipients of tests and treatments.

Engaging you in your healing journey by educating you about the disease and showing what you can do helps build a greater sense of control over your life. This is more than "feel good" talk; studies show that people with cancer who are fully engaged with their treatment and have a fighting spirit have better treatment outcomes.

There is no one-size-fits-all protocol in integrative oncology. Rather, your integrative oncologist will take a customized approach to choose the right treatments for you and will take various factors into account, such as the cancer type and stage, your general health status, symptoms, the safety and efficacy of a treatment, and its cost and availability.

Examples of integrative treatments in cancer care include:

- Acupuncture and acupressure
- Aromatherapy (always in consultation with your medical provider)
- Functional medicine assay testing
- Herbal or botanical therapy (always in consultation with your medical provider)
- Journaling
- Meditation, relaxation, guided visualization
- Movement (yoga, tai chi, dance, aerobic exercise)
- Music therapy
- Nutritional supplements (always in consultation with your medical provider)
- Nutritional therapy
- Spirituality

- Targeted apps and devices, such as a food or exercise tracker
- Touch therapies

Integrative oncology does not involve treatments that are unsupported by science. Scientifically unsupported therapies include:

- Alternative medicines and therapies used in place of effective and proven treatments
- Pseudoscience and therapies in which the quality of the science supporting effectiveness is weak or nonexistent
- Unproven or disproven treatments
- Technologies that claim to measure or alter energy fields that science does not recognize to exist

Getting Started

What's the best way to beat cancer?

First, you and your doctor need to attack cancer from every known front, using a combination from among the most effective conventional treatments: surgery, chemotherapy, radiation.

At the same time, it's important to implement lifestyle measures to alter your body's chemistry, creating an environment in which cancer cells can't thrive. In the following chapters, we describe how simple, daily lifestyle choices—the foods you eat, your physical activity levels, the way you handle stress, the chemicals you're surrounded by—can create this environment.

On their own, lifestyle changes won't cure your cancer. They may, however, greatly improve the outcome of your cancer therapy, help reduce treatment side effects, speed your recovery from treatment, and lower your risk of recurrence.

The strategies you integrate into your daily life can have other positive ripple effects as well, such as better energy levels, improved immune defenses, glowing skin, and fewer colds.

Best of all, these strategies empower you to play a key role in your healing journey.

The book is divided into eight sections:

- Make the Most of Your Treatments
- Eat to Beat Cancer
- Boost Your Defense Systems
- Move Your Body
- Manage Weight
- Get Good Sleep
- Clean Up Your Environment
- Heal Your Mind and Spirit

Again, don't try to do everything at once. Add one change at a time, every few days or weeks. For example, you could:

- Start by calming your mind and lowering your stress levels with a variety of body–mind practices or the help of a counselor or psychotherapist (see p. 239).
- Next, review your diet and make any necessary changes. These could include cutting down on empty calories (alcohol; processed foods; foods made with white flour; candy; etc.) and increasing your intake of nutritious foods (see p. 86).
- Next, start taking a daily walk, beginning with 10–15 minutes and extending it to 30 or 40 minutes, eventually walking up steep inclines or while carrying weights (see p. 193).
- Then, take a hard look at the chemicals you use in daily life and reduce your exposure by changing products (see p. 226).

Each additional measure will bolster your defenses against cancer.

The IOE Cancer Risk Assessment Test combines your body measurements and your dietary, sleep, exercise, and stress-management habits, evaluates which cancer-protective behaviors you already do, and highlights others that you could add. Take the test every six weeks to assess how your behavior changes are modifying your cancer risk. Find it at: **integrativeoncology-essentials.com/cancer-health-test.**

Dr. Lawenda's Integrative Oncology Program

As an online resource, the Integrative Oncology Essentials Program (IOEProgram.com) offers everything you need to empower you on your cancer journey and improve your overall health. Options include:

- A self-paced course with deeper dives into this book's content
- One-on-one consultations with Dr. Lawenda via phone and video conferencing
- Functional medicine lab tests for blood panels, microbiome health, micronutrient assessment, and many more
- The IOE Cancer Risk Assessment Test to improve your ability to prevent and fight cancer
- A community forum to exchange support and ideas with others
- Current articles by Dr. Lawenda on cancer-related topics and research

Visit **IOEProgram.com** to learn more and get started.

Personalized Nutrition & Lifestyle Coaching with Conner

Need help adopting a nutritious, delicious diet and habits that work for your lifestyle and cancer profile? Sign up for Conner's individual and group coaching services at **modernmediterranean.com**. On this website you'll find recipes, articles, and more.

Chapter 2

Make the Most of Your Treatments

Your doctor has delivered the verdict: you have cancer. Understandably, you're in a state of shock.

Now, you can do one of two things:

1. Sign up for treatment at your local cancer center and follow the recommended treatment plan; or
2. Accept the treatments you've been offered and determine additional strategies that empower you to play an active role in your healing journey.

There's certainly nothing wrong with going the first route; most cancer centers will take excellent care of you, and their highly trained oncology professionals—surgeons, radiation oncologists, medical oncologists, nurses, etc.—will apply the best science available to help get you better.

Indeed, some people don't *want* to play an active part in their cancer treatment; they feel overwhelmed by the countless options and prefer one trusted doctor to make the key decisions about their treatment. We fully respect this choice.

If, on the other hand, you want to understand what's happening in your body and make informed choices about your health, we encourage you to pursue the second route. No one knows your body as well as you do, and being an active participant in your treatment can be empowering and life-affirming.

Here's how to get started.

Knowledge Is Power

Learn everything you can, scary though this may be. The more you know, the less room there is for guesswork and anxious rumination.

But don't just search online for terms like "cancer" and "breast"; that's a recipe for confusing and unreliable results. Instead, start with reputable, established organizations such as the American Cancer Society, the American Institute for Cancer Research, or Cancer Research UK for information that's based on the latest scientific research. Also, try government agencies, such as the National Institutes of Health, and renowned cancer treatment centers, such as MD Anderson and Memorial Sloan Kettering.

Dig even deeper by consulting PubMed (**pubmed.gov**), a free online library of peer-reviewed articles published in reputable medical journals. Don't be intimidated by the technical tone; anyone can learn to read them (maybe you can ask a friend or relative with a science background to show you how to read a science article). If a full article requires a fee, ask your local librarian whether they can help you obtain it at reduced cost or free of charge, or email the author and politely request a reprint. Share the articles with your oncologist.

A medical condition like cancer provides a useful opportunity to learn about how your body works. For instance, understanding blood glucose balance and the workings of insulin—and how these may affect your cancer—will help you choose healthier carbohydrates. Realizing how stress affects all body systems will motivate you to manage your stress levels. Knowing how your digestion works will make you appreciate the importance of chewing food thoroughly to maximize nutrient absorption.

Questions, Second Opinions, and Clinical Trials

Ask your doctor as many questions as you have, even if they seem silly. If your oncologist doesn't have the time or inclination to answer them, consult a second or even a third specialist until you understand what's going on and what your options are. Many people feel intimidated by doctors, but remember: They're people, too, and their job is to help you.

Don't feel shy about asking for second opinions from other doctors who specialize in your type of cancer. Oncologists are used to this and many even encourage it. Oncology is a complex and fast-moving medical field where new tests, treatments, and trials are constantly emerging; it would be miraculous for any one doctor to have a definitive answer to every one of your questions.

Participating in a clinical trial gives patients access to innovative treatments that aren't yet available at most cancer centers. But because they're innovative, these treatments may be ineffective or cause undesirable side effects. Usually, experimental therapies are better suited to people who don't respond to most conventional treatments. Talk to your oncologist about options for you.

Grab Your Partner (Your Oncologist)

It's essential to have a care team you trust. If you walk into a doctor's office and feel intimidated, that's a red flag. If your doctor bristles when you ask sensible questions, that's another. And if your doctor discourages you from seeking a second opinion ... time to find another doctor.

You may think that cancer treatment isn't the best time to learn about assertiveness, but in truth, there's no better time to stand up for your needs than when your life is at stake. Learning to advocate for yourself is the alpha and omega of a successful treatment.

Here are 10 ways to boost your confidence when dealing with your medical care team:

1. **Write down questions.** Keep a list of questions in a notebook so when you meet with your doctor or other members of your care team, you remember what you wanted to ask. If your care provider interrupts, wait

for them to finish speaking and then politely resume your list. Jot down answers, or record them.

2. **Keep a record.** Using your smartphone or other digital recorder, record your appointments. This way, you'll be able to recall answers and instructions, and it's easy to share information with your spouse or caregiver. Tell your doctor you'll be recording the session—politely, of course—but don't ask permission. It's your right.
3. **Bring an advocate.** If you feel intimidated or anxious about meetings with your doctor, bring a family member, friend, or patient advocate who can bolster your confidence and help keep the conversation on track.
4. **Respectfully question.** Don't put your doctor on a pedestal. Treat them the same way you would any other professional: with respect, but without giving up all your critical faculties. While they may be a specialist in, say, post-menopausal breast cancer, they may not know much about topics not covered in medical school, such as nutrition or exercise.
5. **Bring up internet info.** Even though a lot of dubious information circulates online, the internet has made it much easier for people to research their symptoms and evaluate treatment options. Rather than using this information to challenge your doctor, use it as a conversation starter. For instance, say, "I read an article on the MD Anderson website that said ___. What do you think of this treatment, and would it be appropriate for me?"
6. **Ask for translations.** It's easy for medical professionals to accidentally slip into technical jargon when talking with patients. If that happens, smile and say: "Would you mind repeating that in plain English, please?"
7. **Maintain your own records.** With the growing prevalence of electronic health records and patient

portals, it's now easy to maintain copies of all your medical records. Make sure you have a printout of every test result and lab report, and keep secure electronic copies on your computer.

8. **Get second opinions.** According to the National Academy of Medicine, one in 20 Americans falls victim to outpatient diagnostic errors. Even if you're comfortable with your doctor's diagnosis, seeking the input of another physician could save you from unnecessary medical costs and stress. Second opinions are available from all major national cancer centers, often via electronic communication rather than in-person visits. (First, make sure your insurance covers it, if cost is a concern.) Learn about second opinions from the American Cancer Society (cancer.org/treatment/finding-and-paying-for-treatment/choosing-your-treatment-team/seeking-a-second-opinion.html).
9. **Catch billing errors.** As many as 80% of medical bills contain errors. Medical bills can be difficult to decipher, but don't give up. Insist on explanations and justifications, even if you meet resistance.
10. **Persevere.** This is your life. Never, ever be afraid to stick up for yourself, even if you're afraid that people will consider you a pest. Don't let anyone discount you. You only have this one life, so go for it!

Shape Your Prognosis

Many people have a blind belief in statistics, especially when presented by a doctor. When you hear your doctor say, "Ninety percent of people with your type of cancer live for another 10 years," that sounds reassuring.

In cases where the prognosis is less positive, however, it can feel downright crushing. It's easy to lose hope and think: "Why bother continuing with treatment and changing lifestyle habits? I've only got a few months left; I might as well enjoy them."

Not so fast! Statistics are just numbers about large groups of people. They're not about you, an individual with a unique set of circumstances. Just because most people with the same type of cancer as yours live for an average length of time after treatment, that doesn't mean you have the same life expectancy.

Why? Because everybody's different! For example, the people you're being measured against may be older than you. Or have other preexisting medical conditions. Or have risk factors that you don't share, such as smoking, heavy drinking, or obesity. Or live in a highly polluted city. Or have a highly stressful job. All these factors influence their ability to continue living healthily, during and after treatment.

In other words, a woman with breast cancer who exercises regularly, eats a Mediterranean diet, gets adequate sleep, and has a strong social support network is likely to have better survival prospects than a woman with the same cancer type and stage but who eats mostly processed foods, leads a sedentary life, suffers from insomnia, and has little social support.

Survival curves are not predetermined; they are dynamic, living entities. And that means you can play an active part in shaping your very own personal survival curve.

Remind yourself (and your doctor): You are not your prognosis. Your health and lifespan are not etched in stone and can change in accordance with the lifestyle changes you make after diagnosis.

Relative or Absolute?

Almost every week you can read about some new and exciting cancer treatment that's infinitely superior to previous therapies. Although this is occasionally true, the benefits of most novel treatments are quite small and often get distorted by data-juggling acts. If results of a treatment or study sound too good to be true, they probably are.

Your oncologist may put some exciting new information this way: "By taking treatment X, your risk of recurrence will be cut by 50%, compared with treatment Y." That sounds compelling, doesn't it?

Before you get too excited, find out whether this outcome differential is expressed in relative or in absolute terms. For while relative difference is what is most often reported, absolute difference is the more useful information.

The relative risk of something happening—for instance, cancer recurrence or treatment side effects—tells you how much more (or less) likely this is to happen in one group compared with another. But relative risk doesn't tell you anything about the *overall likelihood* of any of these things happening; that's what's known as the absolute risk. We can't stress enough how important it is to understand this distinction.

Take this example:

- Cancer recurrence rates are 1% with treatment X and 2% with treatment Y. The relative difference between the two treatments is 50%.
- However, the absolute difference is only 1%. In other words, one out of 100 people experience a recurrence of their cancer with treatment X, and two out of 100 experience a recurrence with treatment Y.
- So, a 50% increase translates into one extra person being helped by treatment X—not a dramatic increase.

Once you find out what the *absolute* difference is between treatment outcomes and side effects, you'll be in a better position to make an informed decision on your options. Ask your oncologist to tell you about absolute risk differences. Don't accept a treatment unless you know this information.

Using Off-Label Drugs

It's increasingly clear that many FDA-approved medications possess powerful anticancer properties. In fact, more than 200 common, generic, noncancer drugs have shown some evidence of anticancer effects. Of these, 50% are supported by relevant human data and 16% by data from at least one positive clinical trial.

Most recently, in a 2020 study, researchers found nearly 50 noncancer drugs, including those initially developed to lower cholesterol or reduce inflammation, that killed some cancer cells while leaving other cells alone.

Instead of waiting years for the FDA to approve new drugs that exploit these anticancer mechanisms, some patients are "repurposing" noncancer prescription drugs to try to improve cancer outcomes.

Physicians already prescribe drugs for off-label use, if it seems reasonable or appropriate. For example, it's not uncommon for doctors to prescribe low doses of beta blockers to help people overcome public-speaking jitters. In such cases, according to the FDA, doctors "have the responsibility to be well informed about the product, to base its use on firm scientific rationale and on sound medical evidence, and to maintain records of the product's use and effects."

People undergoing cancer treatment can repurpose drugs to save both time and money. Generic drugs cost far less than many pharmaceuticals, and they're already FDA-approved as safe, albeit not specifically designed to treat cancer. People with aggressive cancer often feel they don't have the luxury of waiting for clinical trials to prove or disprove the effectiveness of a drug that looks promising in preclinical cancer studies.

However, barriers do exist:

- Many insurance companies won't pay for off-label drug use, because it's considered experimental or investigational
- Off-label drug use may increase legal risk to the healthcare provider, should a patient have an unwanted or bad outcome
- Lack of information about off-label drug use and outcomes may put people at a higher risk for medication errors, side effects, and unwanted drug reactions

If you want to pursue off-label drug use, you first need to acknowledge that:

1. Your cancer is not the same as anyone else's, and your response to any treatment may not be the same as anyone else's; you may develop side effects and toxicities that others may not
2. Taking any drug off-label is an experiment that may improve, worsen, or have no effect on treatment outcomes
3. Interactions with other drugs prescribed by your doctor are possible
4. The labels of many generic drugs are not always accurate in terms of what they do and do not contain

Once you've acknowledged these unknowns, discuss with your oncologist whether they're open to you trying off-label drugs. It is essential that you and your doctor understand and talk about potential side effects, toxicity, and harmful interactions with current medications.

For more information on off-label drugs, visit these recommended resources:

- *How to Starve Cancer*, by Jane McLelland (howtostarvecancer.com)
- ReDO, Repurposing Drugs in Oncology (redo-project.org)
- AntiCancer Fund, "Drug Repurposing" (anticancerfund.org/drug-repurposing)

Tune Up Before Surgery

For people with solid tumors, many cancer treatments begin with surgery to remove as much of the tumor as possible.

Unless surgery must take place immediately, however, take some time to prepare for surgery physically, nutritionally, and emotionally. This process, called prehabilitation (or prehab), can significantly improve the operation's success and speed up your recovery.

By its very nature, surgery causes bodily trauma. Add stress, anxiety, and pain to the mix and you have the perfect storm of inflammation, oxidative stress (free radical production), immune suppression, and insulin resistance. Each of these is linked to worse treatment outcomes, such as extended pain, limited range of motion, and increased risk of infections and blood clots. Prehab is about getting you in the best possible shape for surgery and for later cancer treatment, including chemotherapy and radiation.

It Starts With Food

Your body needs strong nutritional building blocks to heal, fight off infections, and build new tissue after surgery. Ideally, you should start loading up on these nutritional compounds four weeks before surgery and continue for at least four to eight weeks after surgery.

To prepare for surgery, your diet should consist largely of minimally processed fresh foods and as few empty calories (sugar, sodas, white flour, processed food) as possible. Make sure to focus on:

- High-quality protein
- Healthy fats
- Complex carbohydrates like vegetables and fruits (Try to limit your net carbohydrates to 50–100 grams/day. "Net carbs" refers to carbs that are absorbed from the gut into the bloodstream. To calculate the net carbs in whole foods, subtract the fiber from the total number of carbs.)

If you feel you can't meet all of your nutritional needs through food alone, consider adding supplements to shore up your nutrient reserves ahead of surgery. Consult with a nutrition professional or integrative doctor to find out which supplements would best suit your needs. (Please note that some nutrients have blood-thinning effects and shouldn't be taken before surgery. Always consult your doctor before taking nutritional supplements.)

Ahead of surgery and immediately afterward, you can boost your nutritional reserves with high-quality protein powders that provide the essential amino acids your body needs to heal wounds, rebuild tissues, and support the immune system. Simply mix the powder into a glass of water or blend it into a smoothie each day.

To make eating more vegetables and fruits easier, drink them as smoothies. Make your own by combining a variety of fresh or frozen produce each day, which provide essential micronutrients and important anticancer compounds. (See Conner's website, **modernmediterranean.com**, for recipes.)

If you don't have the energy or appliances to make fresh smoothies, try powdered green drinks made from dried whole plants or extracts of grasses, seeds, nuts, fruits, and vegetables. Although they're not as ideal as "real foods," these powders can be a rich source of micronutrients and prebiotics.

If you have trouble controlling your blood glucose (e.g., you have type 2 diabetes or pre-diabetes), try to get it under the best control possible before surgery, either through dietary changes or with the help of medication. Studies show that stress and inflammation from surgery makes insulin less effective, leading to elevated blood sugar levels during and after surgery. This in turn increases the risk of postoperative complications.

Get Calm

Did you know that stress can slow wound healing, impair your immune system, increase inflammation, and cause postoperative pain? Numerous studies have found that people who prepare before surgery with guided imagery and meditation heal faster, have fewer complications, and experience less anxiety and postoperative pain than those who don't. Start a stress-reduction program at least one to two weeks before surgery.

To help calm preoperative fear and anxiety:

- Ask your friends, family, and oncology team for emotional support.

- Ask your care team for written materials and videos on the surgical procedure.
- Use relaxation techniques such as meditation, hypnosis, or guided visualization to prepare your mind for surgery. Check out *Prepare for Surgery*, Heal Faster (healfaster.com), one of our favorite pre-surgery mind-preparation tools. Meditation apps like Headspace and Calm can be very helpful as well.
- Try cognitive behavioral therapy to give you tools to cope with ruminating thoughts or concerns. (Your cancer center may have a CBT practitioner onsite, or should be able to refer you to one.)
- Get more sleep. In the weeks and days before your procedure, aim for seven to eight hours of sleep every night. Sleep is essential for reducing inflammation and stress hormones. (See p. 213 for tips to help you sleep better.)

Get a Baseline Lymphedema Assessment

If you're going to have surgery to the breast, arm, or leg, you could be at risk for a condition called lymphedema. This chronic condition occurs when the body cannot adequately drain lymph fluid from the tissues. It's a common cancer-treatment-related side effect.

Discuss lymphedema risk with your surgeon and get a baseline assessment of your potentially affected body area before surgery so you and your care team can watch for and follow any changes that may occur over time. A certified lymphedema therapist (CLT) can take a baseline measurement of your limbs and educate you about arm or leg care during and after treatment.

If your cancer center doesn't have a lymphedema specialist onsite, ask your doctor for a referral, or consult the Lymphatic Education & Research Network website, lymphaticnetwork.org. Early detection and treatment are of the utmost importance, because the sooner it's diagnosed, the greater your chances of effectively treating lymphedema.

Read This Before Using Opioid Pain Relief

It's important to manage pain during cancer treatments because uncontrolled pain leads to systemic stress and inflammation, both of which are driving factors in cancer progression. Opioids may not always be the best choice, however, and should be used only when other, non-opioid pain therapies are not effective enough.

Many studies report that the use of opioids can suppress the immune system, because they activate the sympathetic nervous system, which generates stress hormones. That's bad for your cancer because:

- Most cancer cells have stress hormone receptors on their surface; when stimulated, these receptors can promote cancer growth
- Stress hormones can also suppress white blood cells' ability to identify and destroy cancer cells
- Opioids can stimulate angiogenesis (the development of new blood vessels that tumors need to grow)

Although much more research is needed to clearly define the risks of opioid use during cancer treatment, many studies associate it with:

- A greater risk of cancer recurrence and metastases
- Suppressed immunity, which increases infection risk and impairs anticancer immune cell activity

Talk to your doctor about alternatives to opioids, such as anticonvulsants, antidepressants, regional pain blocks, neuromodulation, intrathecal drug delivery, cannabinoids, and numerous complementary therapies (acupuncture, aromatherapy, etc.).

While it's worth considering the data and alternative pain management approaches, don't refuse opioids if they are the most effective therapies for managing your pain.

You Don't Have to Be a Hero

Have you ever noticed the paramilitary vocabulary often used about cancer? People describe cancer as an invader, an enemy, or a formidable foe. The person undergoing cancer treatment is described as heroic, a warrior, battling bravely, fighting for their life, kicking cancer's butt, determined to crush cancer, or otherwise engaged in mortal combat with the disease.

But many people with cancer don't experience their illness as a heroic battle. In the moving article "Having cancer is not a fight or a battle," about cancer language in *The Guardian* in April 2014, British doctor and cancer patient Kate Granger wrote:

> "In my world, having cancer is not a fight at all. It is almost a symbiosis where I am forced to live with my disease day in, day out. Some days cancer has the upper hand, other days I do. I live with it and I let its physical and emotional effects wash over me. But I don't fight it. After all, cancer has arisen from within my own body, from my own cells. To fight it would be 'waging a war' on myself. I have submitted myself to [chemotherapy] gently, and somewhat reluctantly, taking whatever each day had to throw at me. I certainly didn't enter the process 'with all guns blazing.'"

There's a reason patients, doctors, and friends use this kind of put-'em-up language. It's meant to be positive, evoke support, and encourage the person not to give up.

But what about the flip side of that conversation? What about someone who "loses" their "fight" against cancer? Someone who has "succumbed"? Were they weak? Would they have "made it" if they had "fought harder"?

For many people undergoing cancer treatment, the fighting language creates pressure to be strong and combative and to not show feelings of fear, sadness, and grief. Warrior metaphors may prevent you from being honest with friends and family. And that can cause loneliness and isolation.

If you find the warrior language supportive and helpful, then use it and encourage others to use it, too. But if it makes you uncomfortable, it's OK to explain to others how you'd prefer to talk about cancer. Don't be someone you don't want to be, be it a hero, victim, or anything in between. You might want to talk with a psychotherapist, counselor, spiritual guide, or hospital chaplain to explore your own thoughts about your illness and how you want to communicate them to the rest of the world.

Prepare for Side Effects

You may well have met, or seen images of, people going through cancer treatment who've lost their hair, appear gaunt and weak, and struggle with gastrointestinal problems like nausea and diarrhea. As you embark on your own treatment, you may think that all this and more awaits you.

To be sure, undergoing cancer treatment is no cakewalk and can take a heavy physical and emotional toll. Some side effects kick in right away, others appear a little later, and some can last long beyond the official end of your treatment.

Preparing for cancer treatment (prehabilitation, discussed on p. 19) can help reduce side effects. Moreover, each person is biochemically unique. While some people suffer severe side effects, others sail through treatment with only a few moments of discomfort. So, go into treatment with an open mind and don't automatically expect the worst.

The following section details complementary approaches that can help limit the most common side effects from cancer treatments (listed in alphabetical order). While these approaches are based on scientific evidence and our own clinical experience, always tell your cancer care team about any complementary treatments you're considering to avoid any potential negative interactions between conventional and alternative treatments.

1. Blood Clots (Thrombosis)

A blood clot can be triggered by tumors that compress blood vessels and slow blood flow. Some cancer drug therapies and radiation therapy can cause inflammation and injure blood vessel walls, a setup for thrombosis.

Emergency treatment may include clot-busting drugs, called thrombolytics, or interventional procedures to remove the blood clot (thrombectomy). In a non-emergency situation, your doctor may prescribe blood-thinning medications or antiplatelet drugs.

Ask your doctor whether you have risk factors for blood clots.

Adopt habits for good circulation to reduce your risks:

- Move your legs frequently while you're sitting (very important on long flights)
- Exercise regularly: at least 30 minutes of moderate aerobic exercise, five days per week
- Maintain a healthy weight
- Stop smoking and avoid secondhand exposure
- Reduce your stress levels
- Wear loose-fitting clothes, stockings, socks
- Wear compression stockings, if your doctor prescribes them
- Stay well-hydrated

Consider baby aspirin. A low dose of aspirin daily may cut risk of developing blood clots by 40%.

Anti-clotting nutrients:

- Instead of low-dose aspirin, eat foods that have high salicylate content (aspirin's active ingredient), which includes many fruits, vegetables, spices, herbs, and beverages
- Vitamin E helps to thin blood; vitamin-E-rich foods include nuts, cold-pressed nut and seed oils, avocado, oats, and wheat germ

- Omega-3 fatty acids also help to thin blood; they're found in oily fish, flaxseed, sunflower seeds, green leafy vegetables
- Curcumin, found in the spice turmeric; it has anticoagulant properties and is widely used in Indian food
- Polyphenol-rich foods: brightly colored fruits, vegetables and berries, olive oil, green and black teas, unsweetened cocoa; polyphenols may help reduce the platelet aggregation process (the clumping together of platelets in the blood), thereby preventing the formation of blood clots
- Garlic, onions, and tomatoes have been shown to reduce platelet aggregation

Explore supplements. Talk to your doctor about foods and supplements that reduce blood clotting:

- Ginkgo biloba
- Rutin (a plant flavonoid)
- Danshen Compound Tablet (a traditional Chinese medicine formula; ask a Traditional Chinese Medicine practitioner with experience in working with people who have cancer)
- Nattokinase (a fermented soybean product)

Always discuss your bleeding risk with your healthcare providers before taking any supplements or consuming large amounts of anti-clotting foods. This is particularly important if you're taking blood-thinning medications (e.g., warfarin, heparin), have had past bleeding problems, have recently had surgery, or if you're scheduled for an upcoming surgery.

Should You Avoid Vitamin K?

No. Not only are the three K vitamins (K1, K2 and K3) essential for healthy blood clotting and strong bones, they may also have cancer-protective effects.

However, vitamin K1 poses a dilemma for some people with cancer. You may be told to eat lots of green vegetables, because these are rich in anticancer compounds, but these very foods are high in vitamin K1, which promotes clotting. If you're taking a blood thinner, such as warfarin, this can cause problems.

Certain nutrients can make warfarin less effective, and one of these is vitamin K. This doesn't mean you have to avoid vitamin-K-containing foods completely, but it's important to be consistent in how much vitamin K you get daily. If you are taking warfarin, limit your daily intake of vitamin K1 to 90 mcg/day for women or 120 mcg/day for men.

Over to You: Blood Clot Prevention Action Plan

- Enhance your blood circulation by moving regularly; avoid prolonged sitting
- Manage your stress; chronic stress and anxiety have been shown to increase coagulation and raise the risk of developing blood clots
- Avoid constricting clothing, but wear compression stockings if your doctor recommends them
- Consider taking low-dose aspirin; discuss this with your doctor
- Eat a diet rich in oils, vegetables, fruits, herbs, and spices that reduce blood clotting—a plant-based eating pattern like the Mediterranean diet, for instance; if you take blood-clotting drugs, discuss with your doctor which foods you need to limit

2. Bone Loss

Several factors cause cancer treatments to raise your risk of bone loss and fractures. Ask your doctor to assess your bone health before you begin treatment, and use these tips to protect your bones.

Work with weights. Aim to do at least 30 minutes of moderate, weight-bearing exercise—which forces you to work against gravity—five to seven days per week. Examples include weight training, walking, hiking, jogging, climbing stairs, tennis, yoga, and dancing.

Don't smoke. According to the National Institutes of Health, there is a direct relationship between tobacco use and decreased bone density.

Manage stress. Stress causes your body to excrete calcium, magnesium, and iron through urine, which can lead to bone mineral loss. Moreover, stress hormones such as cortisol block your body's absorption of calcium. See p. 239 for stress-relieving strategies.

Vibrate. Some research shows that standing on a vibration plate device, which creates low-magnitude, whole-body vibration, can slow bone loss.

Eat well. Key dietary factors for bone health include:

- **Vitamin D.** It increases calcium absorption, maintains bone density, and reduces systemic inflammation. Have your blood levels of vitamin D tested to see if they are adequate.
- **Calcium.** The Institute of Medicine recommends that women younger than 50 and men younger than 71 consume 1,000 mg of this mineral; women over age 50 and men over age 71 should get 1,200 mg. Get as much of your daily calcium as possible from food, such as green leafy vegetables, nuts and seeds (and their butters, like almond butter and tahini), bone-in canned sardines and salmon, tofu, and dairy.
- **Vitamin K2.** Needed by the body to help it properly utilize dietary calcium, it's found in egg yolks, butter, cheese, meat, liver, and fermented foods.
- **High-quality protein (such as lean chicken, beef, pork, tuna, dairy foods, preferably fermented, like yogurt).** Lysine, an amino acid found mostly in animal protein, helps the body absorb and conserve calcium and to form collagen, which makes up the bone matrix.

- **Steady blood sugar.** When blood sugar levels drop too low, the adrenal glands produce cortisol; chronically elevated cortisol reduces the activity of bone-building cells, lowers bone-mineral density, and increases fracture risk. Don't skip meals, and eat small, healthy snacks between meals if you're feeling hungry.
- **Limit sugars and grains.** Sugar-sweetened and grain-based foods such as pasta, bread, and cereal can weaken bones. Limit grains. Use small amounts of natural sweeteners, like maple syrup, if necessary.
- **Limit high-oxalate foods.** Oxalate (oxalic acid) blocks calcium absorption. Foods high in oxalate include spinach, rhubarb, certain beans, and beet greens.
- **Watch your sodium intake.** High salt intake can cause your body to excrete calcium. Keep your daily sodium intake under 2,400 mg.
- **Limit caffeine.** Caffeine in coffee, tea, and soft drinks may contribute to bone loss by decreasing calcium absorption. Drinking more than two cups a day may accelerate bone loss.
- **Limit alcohol.**

Soak legumes. Beans, lentils, and chickpeas are high in calcium, but they also contain phytates, substances that interfere with calcium absorption. Soaking dry beans in water for 12–24 hours, draining and rinsing them, and then cooking them in fresh water significantly reduces phytate levels. Soaking, sprouting and cooking also reduces the lectin content in legumes; lectins are compounds that can hinder nutrient absorption and irritate the gut lining.

Drink bone broth. Chicken and beef bones contain bone-building collagen and minerals. Use bone broth in soups, stews, and grain dishes.

Over to You: Bone Loss Action Plan

- Begin a resistance exercise routine—even a few squats and lunges a day are a great start; ask a physical therapist to design a suitable resistance training routine for you
- Quit smoking
- Manage stress (see p. 239)
- Try vibration therapy; ask your doctor or physical therapist to recommend a device
- Improve nutrition (make one change, then a second, then a third)
- Soak dry beans before cooking
- Chug some bone broth and use it in soups and to cook grains

3. Cancer-Related Fatigue (CRF)

Up to 80% of all people treated with chemotherapy or radiation therapy experience cancer-related fatigue (CRF). The National Comprehensive Cancer Network defines CRF as "a distressing, persistent, subjective sense of physical, emotional, and/or cognitive tiredness or exhaustion ... that is not proportional to recent activity and interferes with usual function."

CRF can persist for weeks to months following treatments. For many people, CRF is even more distressing than pain, or nausea and vomiting.

Get a CRF assessment. The assessment of CRF requires a focused history and physical exam to evaluate potential causes. Your doctor will check:

- Cancer status—progression or recurrence can manifest with fatigue
- Medications—many medications, supplements, and their interactions can cause fatigue; changing doses,

timing, or specific medication to an alternative drug may help
- Contributing factors—these include pain, emotional distress, sleep disturbances, anemia, malnutrition, activity level, alcohol or substance abuse, and other medical conditions and treatment side effects

Practice sleep hygiene. Sleep disturbances, including sleeping too much, insomnia, or disrupted sleep, affect 30–75% of people with cancer. CRF can worsen with poor sleep hygiene, such as:
- Deviating from a regular sleep schedule
- Napping during the daytime
- Consuming alcohol, caffeine, or high-sugar foods before bed

See p. 213 to learn how to create a conducive sleep environment.

Check nutrition. Speak with a nutrition professional to evaluate any weight changes, assess whether you're eating enough food and nutrients, identify any fluid and electrolyte imbalances, and manage other contributing symptoms (nausea, vomiting, loss of appetite, mucositis, diarrhea, constipation).

Address other side effects. Use the tips throughout this book to address other cancer treatment side effects—anemia, pain, heart failure from chemotherapy, hypothyroidism from radiation therapy to the neck, low testosterone from chemotherapy and radiation therapy, etc. Also, pay attention to effects from noncancer-related medical conditions. This can significantly improve symptoms of CRF.

Exercise. Studies have found that light to moderate intensity aerobic exercise, such as walking, yoga, and qigong, helps reduce CRF symptoms in most people. See p. 193 for more on exercise.

Try light therapy. When you don't get enough light exposure during the day (particularly in the morning), melatonin levels rise and serotonin levels fall. This hormonal disruption can cause sleeping difficulties, fatigue, and depression. Researchers have found that when people are exposed to a bright white light, they feel less depressed, have more energy and sleep better. That's why light therapy boxes are sometimes used to treat fatigue, depression, and circadian disruption.

A light box device shines a full-spectrum white light onto the eyes of the user. For best results, it should be used for 30–90 minutes each morning, within 30 minutes of waking. The most effective devices emit light in a similar spectrum to the sun (without the harmful UV waves); look for one that shines most of its light in the wavelength range of 460 nanometers (blue light) to 550 nanometers (green light).

Ask your doctor or mental health provider if light therapy is a good option for you. Some insurance companies cover light therapy purchases when applicable documentation by physicians is provided.

Explore cognitive behavioral therapy. Cognitive behavioral therapy (CBT) is a type of psychotherapy that helps people understand the thoughts and feelings that influence their behaviors, and develop skills to cope. In one study, investigators found that CBT reduced severe CRF symptoms by 30%. Ask your cancer center to refer you to a CBT therapist.

Modulate your stress response. Increasing relaxation and reducing stimulation of the hypothalamic pituitary axis (HPA) (the interplay between the hypothalamus, pituitary gland, and adrenal glands, which play an important role in the stress response) can improve CRF. Techniques to do this include acupuncture, mindfulness-based stress reduction (MBSR), cognitive-based stress reduction, muscle relaxation, music therapy, counseling, social support, hypnosis, biofeedback, therapeutic massage, and yoga.

Check out meds and supplements. Talk to your care providers about pharmacologic interventions. Psychostimulants such as methylphenidate and modafinil have been shown to be effective and well-tolerated in multiple

CRF studies. Supplements such as L-carnitine, ginseng, ginger extract, and omega-3 fatty acids are also reportedly effective for CRF, although results may vary. Ask your doctor whether these are safe for you.

Over to You: Cancer-Related Fatigue Action Plan

- Ask your doctor for a CRF assessment
- Optimize your sleep (see p. 213)
- Evaluate your diet—are you getting enough calories and nutrients?
- Do some light to moderate exercise, ideally daily
- Ask your doctor about light therapy
- Manage stress; explore cognitive behavioral therapy (CBT)

4. Cancer Related Cognitive Impairment (a.k.a. "Chemo Brain")

For many years, the medical establishment hotly disputed the idea that chemotherapy impairs brain function. Now, however, there's not a shred of doubt that "chemo brain" (also known as CRCI, cancer-related cognitive impairment) is a real medical condition.

The most common symptoms relate to problems with cognition, memory, concentration, processing speed, alertness, energy levels, and mood (increased stress, anxiety, and depression). These effects can impair decision making, multitasking, reading comprehension, conversation flow, and word retrieval.

Many of the most common anticancer drugs cause both acute and chronic changes in brain structure and function. This may be due to drug-induced toxicity of critical brain cells, as well as inflammation caused by some chemotherapy drugs. Chemotherapy can also cause changes in brain tissues' glucose metabolism, resulting in impaired brain function.

While drugs can cause CRCI, there may also be other factors at play. One study discovered, for instance, that nearly one-fourth of the cancer patients experienced cognitive impairment even before starting chemotherapy, possibly due to increased levels of inflammatory molecules associated with cancer. The stress and anxiety that come with a cancer diagnosis and fears of the impending treatment may also contribute to CRCI symptoms.

The vast majority of cancer survivors eventually recover—fully or partially—from CRCI, or they find ways to live with it. The key is to start by reducing the inflammation in your brain and body.

Shift to a nutrient-dense diet. Eat as many anti-inflammatory vegetables, fruits, oils, raw nuts, herbs, and spices as you can—ideally at every meal. The Mediterranean diet is one example of this type of diet. Turn to p. 86 for more.

Move. Get at least 30 minutes per day of moderate-intensity exercise. (See p. 193)

Meditate daily. (See p. 248)

Ask about anti-inflammatory supplements. In addition to a Mediterranean diet, you may wish to supplement with omega-3 fatty acids (especially if you rarely eat oily fish), curcumin, or low-dose aspirin. Small studies have shown benefits in both memory and cognition with various natural products, such as brahmi, ginkgo, Panax ginseng, alpha-lipoic acid, and lion's mane mushroom. Ask your doctor whether you can safely take these.

Get regular, restful sleep. Your brain cannot function optimally unless it gets seven to eight hours of sleep every night to rest and recuperate. If you're having trouble falling asleep or staying asleep, meditation can help. (See p. 248) Optimizing your circadian rhythm can also improve sleep. (See p. 213)

Reduce environmental toxins. Pay attention to your personal care products, household cleaning products, and chemical residues in food. Avoid alcohol and tobacco, and drink pure water. Learn more about reducing toxins on p. 226.

Explore mind-body therapies. Many ancient healing traditions believe that the body's flow of vital energy (called "qi" in Chinese medicine and "prana" in Ayurveda) promotes wellness and health, while imbalances or disruptions of this energy create illness.

For people experiencing chemo brain, commonly used mind-body practices for improving and balancing energy may be helpful:

- Acupuncture
- Qigong
- Massage
- Tai chi
- Yoga
- Brain games, such as crossword puzzles, Sudoku, mahjong

Talk to a neuropsychologist. If you've tried self-help techniques and are still troubled by CRCI, get an evaluation from a neuropsychologist. These doctors can identify problems such as depression, anxiety, fatigue, and medication issues; they'll also identify your areas of strength and where you could use some help. A neuropsychologist may suggest cognitive rehabilitation, often using a technique called cognitive behavioral therapy, which has been shown to improve cognition, memory, and other executive brain functions.

Over to You: Cancer-Related Cognitive Impairment Action Plan

- Eat an anti-inflammatory diet; work with a nutritionist or dietitian if you need help getting started (see p. 175, and chapter 3, pp. 86–172)
- Move daily (see p. 193)
- Meditate (see p. 248)
- Prioritize sleep (see p. 213)
- Try a mind-body therapy (see pp. 244–257)

5. Constipation

Constipation—infrequent or difficult passage of hard stool—can cause significant pain and discomfort. It's a frequent side effect of cancer treatment and can be caused by pain medicines, poor fluid intake, lack of activity and generalized weakness, ignoring the urge to move your bowels, low-fiber diets, or simply not eating much food.

A sluggish thyroid gland and chronic stress may also cause constipation; discuss this with your doctor. If you experience constipation, it's important to discuss this with your cancer care team to make sure it's not caused by a serious medical issue, such as stool impaction or tumor blockage. To help relieve constipation:

Drink more. Dehydration can cause constipation, so drink enough fluids. As a crude rule of thumb, drink half your body weight (in lbs) as fluid oz. For example, if you weigh 150 lbs, drink 75 fl oz a day. A good gauge of adequate hydration is the color of your urine: it should be very pale yellow. Dark yellow or light brown urine indicates dehydration.

Some studies have found sparkling water to be more effective than tap water at relieving constipation. Avoid flavored and artificially or sugar-sweetened soda. Other fluids, like tea, coffee, herbal tea, and broth or soup are also hydrating, though slightly less so than water. In the winter, it may be easier to drink water if you warm it to body temperature.

Eat more fiber. Dietary fiber can increase the bulk and consistency of bowel movements, making them easier to pass. In general, fiber falls into two categories:

- **Insoluble:** Found in wheat bran, vegetables, and whole grains, insoluble fiber adds bulk to your stools and can help them pass more quickly and easily through your digestive system.
- **Soluble:** Found in chia, flax, and psyllium seeds (buy organic psyllium to avoid pesticide and heavy metal

residues), oat bran, barley, nuts, seeds, beans, lentils, peas, and some fruits and vegetables, soluble fiber absorbs water and forms a gel-like substance that softens stools and improves consistency.

To prevent constipation, consume both soluble and insoluble fibers. (If you are prone to gas and bloating, get more soluble than insoluble fiber.) The total recommended fiber intake per day is about 25–30 grams for women and 35–40 grams for men. You can track your fiber intake with a food-journaling app, such as Cronometer.

The foods that contain the most fiber include:

- Beans (white & black)
- Lentils
- Avocados
- Chickpeas
- Bulgur
- Raspberries (raw)
- Collard greens
- Artichokes
- Winter squash
- Sweet potatoes
- Kiwis
- Chia seeds

Exercise. Studies show that exercise, especially walking and yoga (see p. 245), can significantly reduce constipation. (This article features yoga poses for the relief of constipation: medicalnewstoday.com/articles/327086)

Drink coffee. Coffee, especially when it contains caffeine, stimulates digestive system muscles, which in some people produces an urge to empty the bowels. Coffee also may contain small amounts of soluble fiber and polyphenols (beneficial plant compounds) that help prevent constipation by improving the balance of your gut bacteria (see p. 179). Organically grown coffee is best; many brands of conventionally grown coffee are heavily treated with pesticides, herbicides, and fungicides.

Eat fermented foods. People who have chronic constipation frequently have imbalanced gut bacteria. Eating foods that contain beneficial bacteria (probiotics) may help restore a healthier microbial balance. Probiotics may also relieve constipation by increasing the frequency of bowel movements and improving stool consistency.

Probiotic foods include fermented foods like yogurt, kefir, sauerkraut, and kimchi, which contain live, friendly bacteria. Or try a probiotic supplement; take it daily for at least four weeks to see if it has any beneficial effects. (Talk to your doctor before taking any supplement.)

Add prebiotics. Certain fibers found in plant foods nourish the friendly bacteria in your gut, which can improve digestive function; these are called prebiotics. Some prebiotics have been shown to help increase the frequency of bowel movements and make stools softer. Foods that are high in prebiotic fiber include garlic, onions, and bananas.

Inulin, a soluble fiber found in many plants (asparagus, chicory root, garlic, Jerusalem artichoke, jicama), serves as a great prebiotic for gut bacteria. Inulin supplementation has been shown to increase intestinal flora diversity, relieve constipation, promote weight loss, and improve blood sugar control. Consider taking 1–3 tsp of inulin powder mixed into a tall glass of water every day.

Boost your digestive enzymes. Digestive enzymes, made by the pancreas, act on specific molecules within foods to break them down. Not producing enough of these enzymes occurs commonly after gallbladder and pancreatic surgery and may develop naturally as you get older. This can cause digestive problems, including constipation.

You can take digestive enzyme capsules with your meals to substitute for the lack of natural enzyme production. A nonprescription lactase supplement (such as Lactaid) can help people manage lactose intolerance, and an alpha-galactosidase supplement (such as Beano) may reduce gas and bloating if you have a hard time digesting beans. Pineapple contains a natural digestive enzyme called bromelain—also a powerful anti-inflammatory compound—so a little fresh pineapple after meals may help.

Manage magnesium. The mineral magnesium controls muscular contractions. People with low magnesium may experience constipation, because the muscles that are supposed to push food through their digestive tube are sluggish.

To eat more magnesium, increase your intake of magnesium-rich foods: legumes, nuts, seeds, green leafy vegetables, whole grains and—yes!—dark chocolate. A supplement may help; magnesium citrate, for instance, is a popular home remedy against constipation.

An Epsom salts bath can also be effective. Epsom salts are made from magnesium sulfate; while bathing, your body absorbs some magnesium through the skin (it's also very relaxing and can improve sleep). Use one-and-a-half cups (12 oz) of Epsom salts in a standard bathtub. Do not take Epsom salts baths if you're pregnant, have exposed cuts or burns, are severely dehydrated, or have heart disease.

Avoid dairy and/or gluten. Sometimes an intolerance to dairy or gluten-containing foods can cause constipation. Try removing these from your diet for two weeks to see if this improves your symptoms. Be sure to replace the dairy in your diet with other calcium-rich foods.

Head for the drugstore. If none of the above help, ask your doctor to recommend pharmaceutical agents to address constipation. Categories include:

- Stool softeners
- Stimulants
- Osmotic agents
- Opioid antagonists
- Rectal products

Over to You: Constipation Action Plan

- Stay well hydrated
- Consume adequate fiber (track your meals using the Cronometer app for a few days to see how much fiber you're eating)
- Move daily; special yoga poses may help
- Drink coffee (caffeinated coffee has the strongest effect on intestinal activity, but even decaf can stimulate bowel movements)
- Eat foods containing probiotics and prebiotics every day; supplement if necessary
- Eat foods containing digestive enzymes, or take an enzyme supplement
- Eat foods rich in magnesium and/or supplement; an Epsom salts bath provides magnesium and relaxation
- Ask your doctor for pharmaceutical agents to relieve constipation

6. Diarrhea

Diarrhea is common in people undergoing cancer treatment. It's important to identify what's causing it, so it can be addressed quickly, before you become dangerously dehydrated or lose too much weight. Causes include:

- Radiation to the abdomen
- Surgical removal of bowel (small intestine, colon, or rectum)
- Chemotherapy drugs
- Medicines, such as magnesium-based antacids, laxatives, and other drugs
- Antibiotics
- Spicy foods, deep-fried foods, and hot liquids, especially after abdominal surgery

- Food sensitivities or allergies
- Alcohol, caffeine, and enteral nutrition supplements
- Stomach flu (gastroenteritis), diverticulitis, or irritable bowel syndrome (IBS)
- Digestive enzyme insufficiency
- Adding supplemental fiber to your diet too quickly

Drink 8–12 cups of fluids every day. Diarrhea can quickly make you dehydrated if you don't drink enough. Check the color of your urine: If it's dark instead of pale yellow, you're not drinking enough.

Rice or barley water, fresh vegetable juices (especially carrot and celery), miso broth, or other clear broths can help restore proper fluid and electrolyte balance. To make rice or barley water, add 1 cup raw grains to 1 quart of boiling water and steep for 20 minutes. Strain and drink throughout the day.

Hot fluids (including soups) may make diarrhea worse. Allow hot fluids to cool to room temperature before drinking.

Eat BRAT. The BRAT diet (bananas, (white) rice, applesauce, and dry toast) can help slow down movement in the GI tract. This isn't a very nourishing diet, however, so don't eat it for more than a day or two.

Rice water (from cooking rice in a large volume of water) can also help bind the stools. Bring a quart of water to a boil and add ½ cup white rice; cook for 30 minutes, remove from heat and let the rice settle at the bottom of the pot. With a ladle, scoop off the water and drink two to three times a day until the diarrhea stops.

Get probiotics. Yogurt, kefir, and probiotics taken as powder or in capsules (lactobacillus GG, acidophilus, or bifidobacteria) help maintain the healthy bacteria in your intestines and may alleviate diarrhea. If your immune system is weak, or you're taking immunosuppressive drugs, check with your doctor as to whether probiotics from food or supplements are safe for you.

Eat small, frequent meals. If you struggle with diarrhea, use these meal guidelines:

- Limit high-fiber foods (beans, cruciferous vegetables, leafy greens, whole grains)
- Limit high-fat foods (fried foods, rich desserts, buttery or creamy sauces, oily dishes)
- Avoid alcohol, caffeine, and spicy foods
- Limit milk and other dairy products. Cultured milk products such as yogurt, buttermilk, and hard cheeses may be better tolerated
- Limit use of sugar-free products that contain sorbitol or xylitol; these exacerbate diarrhea

Try herbal infusions. Infusions made with herbs like slippery elm, peppermint, and marshmallow root can help to soothe an inflamed and irritated gut. Health food stores sell herbal teas (in teabags) formulated to soothe irritated digestive tracts, but you can also make herbal teas from scratch.

To make slippery elm tea, pour 2 cups of filtered, just-boiled water over 2 tablespoons of the powder and steep for a few minutes. Slippery elm bark powder can be found in health food stores and online.

Marshmallow root and mint can be combined in a gut-soothing tea: Place 1 tablespoon marshmallow root and 1 tablespoon dried peppermint leaf in a mason jar and cover with 2 cups cold or room-temperature filtered water. Place in the fridge for at least three hours or overnight. Strain and drink cold. Marshmallow root tea can be found in health food stores and online.

Gentle hygiene. Use mild, unperfumed baby wipes to clean the anal area after each bowel movement. Apply a calming, water-repellent ointment to the anal area. Also, log the number and frequency of bowel movements you're having; this will help you and your care team to adjust treatments as needed.

Call your doctor if ...

- You have six or more loose bowel movements a day with no improvement in two days
- You notice blood in or around the anal area or in the stool
- You lose five pounds or more after the diarrhea starts
- You notice new belly pain or cramps for two days or more
- You don't urinate for 12 hours or more
- You are unable to drink liquids for 24 hours or more

Over to You: Diarrhea Action Plan

- Identify the cause of your diarrhea; consult with your doctor
- Drink lots of fluids and ensure you're getting electrolytes (broths, vegetable juices, barley water; add electrolyte powders where necessary, but avoid highly sweetened "sports" drinks)
- Eat the BRAT diet for a day or two (bananas, (white) rice, applesauce, toast)
- Get probiotics from foods and supplements
- Eat small, frequent meals
- Sip soothing herbal infusions

7. Dry Mouth

Dry mouth (xerostomia) is a common side effect from cancer treatments for head and neck cancers. It may manifest as a sticky dry feeling in the mouth; thick, stringy saliva; a dry, tough tongue; dry or cracked lips; mouth sores; and more.

Chemotherapy causes dry mouth by making saliva thicker. This is usually a temporary symptom that clears up two to eight weeks after treatment ends.

Radiation therapy to the head, face, or neck may also cause dry mouth; after treatment ends, it can take six months or longer for the salivary glands to start working again. Some people experience long-term dry mouth, especially if radiation was directed at the salivary glands.

Some drugs, such as diuretics, pain medications, and certain antidepressants, can also cause dry mouth, so discuss with your doctor what might be causing this problem.

Simulate and stimulate saliva:

- Use saliva substitutes and mouth rinses with hyetellose, hyprolose, or carmellose
- Talk to your doctor about medicines that stimulate the salivary glands, such as pilocarpine (Salagen) or cevimeline (Evoxac)
- Stimulate the salivary glands by sucking on sugar-free candy or chewing sugarless gum

Soothe your mouth:

- Breathe through your nose, not your mouth
- Apply coconut oil to your lips to prevent cracking
- Avoid mouthwashes and other dental products that contain alcohol; dry-mouth products are available without a prescription
- Consider acupuncture; some research suggests it can help with dry mouth

Increase moisture with diet:

- Drink plenty of liquids (at least 8 cups a day), both between and with your meals
- Suck on frozen-juice ice cubes or fruit-puree popsicles
- Snack on "moist" foods like melon or cucumbers whenever your mouth feels dry
- Eat fibrous foods that require a lot of chewing, like raw carrots, to spur saliva production
- Use herbs and spices shown to increase saliva, including fennel, ginger, and endive
- Avoid alcohol and caffeine-containing drinks, which can dehydrate the mucous membranes of the mouth
- Avoid dry foods (crackers, bread, cake, cookies)

- Add sauces, dressings, broth, or pureed vegetables and fruits to your foods
- Avoid acidic or spicy foods that can burn your mouth
- Avoid sticky, sugary foods and drinks

Protect your teeth:

- Visit a dentist before starting chemotherapy or radiation therapy to the head and neck. If you need to have teeth removed, get this done before starting treatments so your gums can heal. If you have dry mouth after cancer treatments are over, see a dentist who is experienced in working with cancer patients and survivors.
- Brush your teeth after each meal and at bedtime with a soft-bristle toothbrush and fluoride toothpaste. Soak the brush in warm water to make the bristles even softer.
- Floss gently once a day.
- Rinse your mouth four to six times a day, especially after meals, with a solution of 1/2 teaspoon salt and 1/2 teaspoon baking soda in 1 cup of warm water.
- If you're getting radiation therapy for a head and neck cancer, your dentist may recommend fluoride rinses or gels. Some dentists may also prescribe medicines to increase saliva or rinses to treat mouth infections.

Over to You: Dry Mouth Action Plan

- Drink at least 8 cups of water a day—ideally, more. If you find water boring, flavor it with lemon or lime juice or drink cooled herbal tea or iced tea
- Stock up on moist foods, like melon cubes and cucumber slices
- Invest in a soft toothbrush and delicious toothpaste so dental hygiene feels less like a chore
- Make a quart of salt-and-bicarbonate rinse that you can use to rinse your mouth after meals

8. Hair Loss

Some cancer drugs and doses cause anything from hair thinning to full-body baldness. Talk to your care team about the drugs you'll be taking. They can tell you what to expect. Fortunately, chemo-related hair loss is usually temporary.

Ask about cold cap therapy. What you may not know is that it's possible to preserve your hair, or at least reduce hair loss, by cooling the scalp during chemotherapy infusions.

Cold cap therapy (CCT) involves wearing special caps, frozen to a very cold temperature, during each chemotherapy session—typically 20–30 minutes before the start of each session and up to 90 minutes afterwards, depending on the chemo type. Scalp cooling reduces blood flow to the scalp and the metabolism of chemotherapy in the hair follicles, resulting in reduced hair loss.

For over 40 years, mainly in Europe, people undergoing cancer treatment have used CCT. Cold caps were first approved in the United States in 2015 for breast cancer patients receiving chemotherapy. Now, it's approved for all solid-tumor cancers.

Recent studies indicate that cold cap therapy can prevent hair loss in 10–100% of those who use it, with most studies showing about 50% effectiveness. Results vary due to factors such as the type of chemo drugs, timing and compliance, and proper technique. Only 3–13% of people discontinue CCT because of discomfort, such as headache or dizziness.

There are two main types of CCT devices: manual frozen gel caps and machine cap cooling systems. Cost varies but typically runs from $1,500 to $2,200. Unfortunately, many insurance companies don't cover CCT, but it's definitely worth asking.

CCT isn't a good choice for every type of cancer or chemo treatment, so ask your oncologist. If you get approval, you can rent the manual frozen gel cap devices directly from manufacturers. (The machine cap cooling systems are still not available in most oncology offices.)

Why don't we hear more about CCT in the U.S.? Early CCT technology wasn't very effective. The older CCT caps were not as well-fitting or cold enough, and the regimens were not as rigorous.

Furthermore, some oncologists are concerned that by reducing blood flow (and chemotherapy) to the scalp and skull, CCT might increase the risk of tumors in the scalp and skull, especially in people who have cancers of the blood (leukemia) and lymph (lymphoma).

We believe this risk is overestimated. In women with breast cancer, for instance, the risk of scalp and skull metastases has been shown to be extremely low: 0.04–1%.

Use coping strategies. When hair loss from chemotherapy can't be prevented, use these coping strategies:

- Consider cutting your hair short or shaving your head once hair loss begins
- Use mild, natural shampoos and soft hair brushes
- Avoid blow dryers, curling irons, and other hot styling appliances
- Keep your scalp clean and moisturized
- Protect your scalp from the sun with hats, wigs, or sunscreen
- Be creative: use colorful scarves, turbans, or hats; most cancer centers offer classes where they teach you how to fashion creative headwear; if yours doesn't, watch instructional videos on Headcovers.com's YouTube channel (http://www.youtube.com/c/HeadcoversUnlimited/videos)
- Wear a good-quality wig; check with your insurance company to see if they will help cover the cost

Over to You: Hair Loss Action Plan

- Discuss the pros and cons of cold cap therapy with your oncologist; check that your insurance covers this treatment.
- If hair loss is inevitable, take good care of your scalp and get advice about wigs and head scarves from your cancer center

9. Hot Flashes

Men and women alike may experience hot flashes from taking hormone medications, commonly prescribed for hormone-sensitive cancers, such as breast and prostate cancer. Antidepressants, such as Effexor, may help—although they may have unpleasant side effects of their own. We suggest you start by trying the complementary strategies below to reduce hot-flash frequency and intensity.

Explore complementary therapies. Evidence shows that acupuncture can be equally effective as Effexor at reducing hot flashes, without the antidepressant's nasty side effects. People with hot flashes may benefit from a four-week trial of acupuncture. Meditation, breathing exercises, cognitive behavioral therapy, and hypnotherapy may also help.

Eat a Mediterranean diet. A diet high in vegetables and fruits, and low in sugar and processed oils, has been shown to reduce the incidence of hot flashes in menopausal women by 23%, and may well help relieve androgen-therapy-related hot flashes.

Keep cool. Keep the temperature of your room low (around 65°F). Use sleepwear and sheets made from natural fibers, like organic cotton, linen, or bamboo. Consider using a cooling mattress pad, such as Ooler (chilitechnology.com).

Acupuncture. In addition to relieving hot flashes, acupuncture can help reduce pain, muscle, or joint stiffness, inflammation, stress and anxiety, sleep problems, nausea, dry mouth, and many other common cancer-treatment symptoms.

Acupuncture is based on an elegant and complex system derived from traditional Chinese medicine. Acupuncturists create an individualized combination of acupuncture points based on a diagnostic process that includes a physical exam, medical and lifestyle history, and symptoms.

Acupuncture needles are very thin, stainless steel, sterile, and single-use. Most people do not feel any discomfort. Acupuncture needles are inserted into the top layer of skin only, and rarely cause any bleeding or bruising. You may feel relaxed, energized, or emotional after an acupuncture session; effects vary from person to person.

Select an acupuncturist who has experience with cancer patients and survivors. Ask your oncology providers for a recommendation. Check with your medical insurance carrier; approximately 60–70% of insurance plans cover acupuncture treatments.

Over to You: Hot Flash Action Plan

- Try acupuncture
- Try hypnotherapy (see p. 60)
- Keep cool at night
- Reduce or eliminate sugar and refined carbs, coffee, and alcohol
- Eat a Mediterranean diet rich in vegetables, fruits, and legumes

10. Low Blood Counts

Throughout your treatment, your cancer care team will closely monitor your blood with complete blood count (CBC) tests, which keep an eye on three major types of blood cells:

- **White blood cells (WBC).** These help your immune system fight infection. A low WBC count (leukopenia) leaves your body more vulnerable to infection.
- **Red blood cells (RBC).** Red blood cells' ability to carry oxygen throughout your body depends on the amount of hemoglobin in your blood. If your hemoglobin is low (anemia), your body has to work harder to supply oxygen to your tissues, making you feel tired and short of breath. Another RBC test, the hematocrit, assesses the volume of RBCs in your blood. Low hematocrit also indicates anemia.
- **Platelets.** Platelets help your blood to clot. A low platelet count (thrombocytopenia) can make it hard for your body to stop bleeding if you're injured.

Chemotherapy, radiation therapy, and cancers of the blood and bone marrow all cause low blood cell counts. Common treatments include blood transfusions, medications, or stopping or delaying treatment.

Optimize your diet. Because all body cells are made from the foods you eat, eating well supports healthy blood counts or helps improve low ones. To boost your blood, be sure to get enough:

- Protein, the building block of all cells
- Iron, B12, folate, copper, and vitamin A, which boost red blood cell counts
- Iron, B12, folate, and vitamin C, which boost platelet production

Take a gentle walk. Research shows that non-strenuous exercise can increase both red and white blood cell counts. Take daily walks, and bring your partner or a friend in case you feel faint and need help getting back.

Avoid injury. A low platelet count makes even minor abrasions potentially serious. Consider using an electric shaver to avoid nicks. Ask someone else to chop ingredients for recipes. Be gentle when brushing your teeth or blowing your nose.

Minimize germs. Wash your hands frequently, or use liquid hand sanitizer. Stay away from crowds and people who are sick. Have someone else clean the litter box, birdcage, or fish tank. Don't eat raw meat or raw eggs.

Over to You: Low Blood Count Action Plan

- Talk with a nutritionist or dietitian about blood-boosting foods and supplements
- Take a daily walk with a friend
- Use an electric razor
- When cooking, enlist someone to cut up ingredients
- Wash hands often
- Have someone else clean pet stations

11. Lymphedema

Up to five million Americans suffer from lymphedema, a consequence of surgery or radiation therapy to the lymph nodes in the neck, armpit, pelvis, and groin areas, leading to impaired draining of lymph fluid and causing fluid accumulation. Without intervention, lymphedema can lead to progressive swelling, fibrosis, pain, nerve damage, and infection.

Practice prevention. Talk with your surgeon or radiation oncologist about whether your treatments could place you at higher risk of lymphedema. A certified lymphedema therapist (CLT) can take a baseline measurement of your limbs and educate you about arm or leg care during and after treatment. Ask your doctor for a referral or consult the Lymphatic Education & Research Network website, lymphaticnetwork.org, to find a practitioner.

Start decongestive therapy. Once lymphedema is diagnosed, treatment should begin quickly. While there are no curative treatments, the sooner decongestive treatment is started, the better the outcomes of reversing the overt clinical symptoms. The goals of treatment are to decrease the excess volume as much as possible and maintain the limb or other affected tissues (i.e., breasts, neck, abdomen, back) at its smallest size.

The most common lymphedema treatment is complete decongestive therapy (CDT), which involves a treatment and a maintenance phase. The treatment phase (daily, for two to four weeks) consists of:

- Inspecting skin and nails to confirm that they are free of any cuts, scratches, areas of irritation, or signs of infection
- Manual lymphatic drainage (MLD), a massage-like technique performed for 30–60 minutes to improve lymphatic flow
- Application of compression bandaging, worn 24/7 during the treatment phase; these apply pressure during movement to stimulate the flow of lymph fluid
- Therapeutic exercise, performed with the compression bandages in place

The maintenance phase is a daily, lifelong, self-care program that includes self-MLD, skin and nail care, compression garments worn during waking hours, compression bandaging at night if necessary, and a home exercise program.

Over to You: Lymphedema Action Plan

- Before you begin cancer treatment, ask your doctor about your lymphedema risk
- Get a baseline assessment from a certified lymphedema therapist (CLT); ask them to show you how to care for your limbs throughout treatment
- Use exercises, bandages, and manual lymphatic drainage throughout treatment and beyond to maintain tissue health; ask your CLT or a specialized physical therapist to guide you

12. Mucositis

Radiation therapy and chemotherapy drugs can trigger a cascade of inflammatory reactions that lead to mucositis, painful sores and ulcers in the mucous membranes of the mouth and throat. Harmful bacteria and fungi then move in to colonize these inflamed tissues, worsening the condition.

With chemotherapy, mucositis can develop throughout the entire gastrointestinal system within five to 10 days of starting therapy and can last for two to four weeks afterward. Radiation-related mucositis only develops when therapy is directed at cancers of the mouth and throat. Typically, the first signs begin about three weeks into treatment, peak a few days after the final session, and can last for several weeks to months after completing treatment.

Once chemotherapy and radiation therapy are no longer stimulating the inflammatory process, the mucous membranes begin healing and the natural flora of oral microorganisms returns to normal.

Notify your healthcare team if you notice worsening sores, white patches, pus, bleeding in the mouth or throat, or a fever greater than 100.4°F.

Practice prevention:

- Get checked. Prior to starting cancer treatments, see a dentist who is experienced in working with people with cancer. You'll be checked for dental and gum disease to determine if you need any urgent treatment before starting chemotherapy or radiation therapy. If you have a dental appliance, your dentist will assess whether it fits properly to avoid irritation to mouth tissues.
- Optimize oral hygiene. Your dentist or hygienist will discuss this in great detail with you before starting cancer treatments.
- Brush your teeth after every meal and floss daily to reduce buildup of the bacteria that can cause plaque and gingivitis. (Do not floss if your platelet count is below 40,000.) Proper technique will help prevent injuring

your gums. See here how to brush (mouthhealthy.org/en/az-topics/b/brushing-your-teeth) and floss (mouthhealthy.org/en/az-topics/f/flossing).

- Use a soft toothbrush and change it every three to four months. Never share a toothbrush, and thoroughly rinse toothbrushes with water after brushing.
- Avoid toothpastes with whitening agents.
- Use a non-alcoholic mouth rinse to further reduce plaque-causing bacteria.
- The Oral Cancer Foundation recommends rinsing your mouth before and after meals and at bedtime with salt water (1 teaspoon of salt dissolved in 1 quart of water), or a salt–baking soda rinse (1/2 tsp of salt and 1–2 tablespoons of baking soda dissolved in 1 quart of warm water).
- Keep lips moist with moisturizers. Avoid Vaseline because the oil base can promote infection.
- Use a humidifier (particularly when sleeping at night).
- If you wear dentures, remove them whenever possible to expose your gums to air. Don't wear loose-fitting dentures, and don't wear dentures if your mouth sores are severe.
- Avoid foods that are spicy, hot, acidic, or coarse.
- Avoid tobacco products.
- Increase your fluid intake.

Try ice. Sucking on ice chips can help reduce mucositis during the administration of certain chemotherapy drugs. Ice helps to reduce the blood flow and perfusion of drugs into mouth tissues during chemotherapy infusion.

Ask about laser therapy. Low-level laser therapy (also known as cold laser therapy, infrared laser therapy, or photobiomodulation therapy) is effective for reducing mucositis risk and severity. Daily laser therapy on the tongue, lips, gums, cheeks, roof, and floor of the mouth helps speed up the cells' rate of repair in the underlying mucous membranes.

This works best if you start at the beginning of chemotherapy or radiation therapy.

If your medical team can't refer you to a cold laser therapist, you'll need to do some research to find a local provider who offers this treatment (for instance, a nearby academic center, chiropractor, integrative medicine provider, radiation oncologist, etc.).

Reduce severity and infection risk:

- Continue maintaining strict oral hygiene to minimize inflammation
- Keep rinsing with salt water (with or without baking soda) or antiseptic rinses; these rinses can help reduce the buildup of thick phlegm and mucous production, a common side effect of treatments.

Use barriers. Mucosal protectants are compounds that form a protective barrier to help reduce the severity of mucositis. They're quite effective and may work even better if started before mucositis sets in. Your doctor can prescribe mucosal protectants.

Nonprescription mucosal protectants include:

- Honey: 1–2 tablespoons, swish and swallow; or add to any warm (not hot) tea
- Slippery elm or marshmallow root tea
- Licorice extracts
- Deglycyrrhizinated licorice (DGL) tablets: Chew one every two hours, as needed

Soothe pain with:

- Mouth rinses with aloe, green tea, chamomile, curcumin, ginger, peppermint
- Benezydamine hydrochloride oral rinse (a topical anti-inflammatory)
- Topical pain relievers (lidocaine, benzocaine, xylocaine)
- Cannabinoids

Eat well:

- Maintain healthy eating; a strong nutritional status is essential to reduce the risk and severity of mucositis (see pp. 86–90)
- Avoid spicy, acidic, or hot foods and liquids, as well as alcoholic beverages
- Eat soft, moist foods, such as soft fresh or stewed fruit, cooked (rather than raw) vegetables, oatmeal, pureed or mashed foods, soups, smoothies, and scrambled eggs
- Choose cold foods and drinks, such as homemade fruit popsicles, frozen fruit-juice ice cubes, or frozen cherries
- Drink through a straw to bypass mouth sores

People who have been treated with radiation therapy to the head and neck or who underwent chemotherapy may develop permanent thinning of the mucous membrane tissues, thickened salivary secretions and/or dry mouth. Late effects can increase the risk of dental caries (cavities), gingivitis (inflammation of the gums), mucosal sensitivity and pain, and diminished taste sensation. Continue to have regular dental checkups after your cancer treatment is over. If you have dental appliances, they may need to be adjusted due to changes in tissue.

Over to You: Mucositis Action Plan

- Prioritize oral hygiene
- Find a cold (low-level) laser therapy practitioner; this is most effective when you start at the beginning of chemo or radiation therapy
- Use mucosal protectants
- Swish with topical pain relievers and mouth rinses
- Eat nutritious, soothing foods

13. Nausea and Vomiting

If vomiting lasts longer than 30 minutes, call your doctor.

Eat wisely:

- Eat small, frequent meals, rather than fewer, larger meals.
- Sip liquids—mainly water and herbal teas—between meals. If you feel very nauseous, sip them slowly, in small spoonfuls. Avoid drinking at mealtimes, which can exacerbate nausea.
- Frequent vomiting can deplete important electrolytes and cause dehydration. Drink water with added electrolyte-balancing powders (available at any drugstore) until the vomiting stops.
- Infuse coarsely chopped raw ginger in hot water and sip it lukewarm, at room temperature, or chilled, perhaps flavored with lemon and a little honey. (Check with your doctor before using ginger.) Or try peppermint tea.
- Ginger taken in capsules (500 mg, twice a day) has been found to significantly reduce the severity of chemotherapy-induced nausea.
- Eat under calm, relaxed conditions. Rest after meals, preferably in a sitting position.
- Eat slowly and chew your food thoroughly.
- If strong flavors or odors turn you off, eat bland foods such as lightly poached chicken breasts or white fish, plain brown rice or pasta, and vegetables such as carrots, sweet potatoes, peas, green beans, or zucchini.
- Avoid eating hard-to-digest foods (fatty, fried, or spicy dishes, for example).

Use pharmaceuticals. Prescriptions for nausea and vomiting can be taken on an as-needed basis, or preventively. Ask your doctor.

Try cannabinoid tincture. Numerous studies report the effectiveness of pharmaceutical synthetic cannabinoid drugs, as well as natural cannabinoids and their extracts. Try a trial of a full-spectrum marijuana extract tincture with a

1:1 THC-CBD ratio, available at most dispensaries. Tinctures can either be applied under the tongue or swallowed. Learn more about cannabis on p. 80.

Learn laser acupuncture. Acupuncture is a highly effective treatment for various cancer-related symptoms, including chemotherapy-induced nausea and vomiting.

One little-known method of acupuncture uses lasers. Recent studies demonstrate that certain low-energy lasers, also called "cold" or "low-level light therapy" lasers, are an effective, noninvasive, painless alternative to needles for stimulating acupuncture points. This technique is an appealing alternative for people with a weakened immune system, bleeding abnormalities, or needle phobia. Laser acupuncture is quite safe, though protective goggles are recommended.

Laser acupuncture—unlike traditional acupuncture using needles—requires no more technical skill than using a laser pointer. Each acupuncture laser comes with instructions on how long the treatments should take per point (typically 15–60 seconds per point). You can find these points on this useful web page: https://pointfinder.org/vomiting/.

The most common acupoints include:

- PC-6 (pericardium 6): on the inside wrist
- SP-6 (spleen 6): above the tip of the inner ankle bone, on the back of the shinbone
- ST-36 (stomach 36): below the kneecap, on the outside, in a depression between the shinbone and leg muscle
- LR-3 (liver 3): on the top of the foot, above where the big toe and the second toe separate; both feet are treated
- LI-4 (large intestine 4): in the muscle belly between the thumb and the index finger; both hands are treated

Practice moxibustion. The ancient Chinese technique called moxibustion involves the use of a rolled herbal "cigar" of dried mugwort, also called moxa. A smoldering moxa is held directly over the skin at specific acupuncture points to stimulate their activity.

Acupuncturists can provide moxibustion treatments, but you can easily practice it yourself whenever you feel a wave of nausea approaching. Moxa rolls are inexpensive and easy to use. Ask an experienced acupuncturist to show you how. The advantage of self-treatment is that you can do this whenever you need it, rather than having to wait for your acupuncture appointment.

Employ body–mind practices:

- Guided imagery can significantly reduce nausea and vomiting. One study showed significant reductions in chemo-induced nausea and vomiting in women with breast cancer using imagery. We particularly like the guided imagery collections by psychotherapist Belleruth Naparstek (healthjourneys.com).
- Hypnosis creates a state of intense attention, willingness, and readiness to accept an idea. It's increasingly used as an adjunct to local anesthetic and can also help alleviate chemotherapy-induced nausea. Unfortunately, hypnotherapy is not regulated in the U.S., but two professional organizations—the National Board for Certified Clinical Hypnotherapists (natboard.com) and the American Society of Clinical Hypnosis (asch.net)—provide certification and can be a good place to find a practitioner. You can also teach yourself self-hypnosis with training from a medical hypnosis specialist (individually or in a group session), or through books, CDs, DVDs, or downloads (for instance, at hypnosisdownloads.com).
- Keep your home well-aired and take gentle walks with deep breathing. Wear loose-fitting clothing.

Over to You: Nausea & Vomiting Action Plan

- If you vomit for more than 30 minutes, call your doctor
- Eat frequent, small, calm, mild-tasting, easy-to-digest meals
- Sip fresh ginger infusions or take ginger capsules
- Discuss anti-nausea medications and/or cannabis with your doctor
- Laser self-acupuncture
- Explore body-mind practices like guided imagery and hypnosis
- Get plenty of fresh air; practice deep breathing

14. Pain and Neuropathy

Pain affects 59% of people undergoing cancer treatment and 64% of those with advanced cancer. Even after treatment is over, 33% of cancer survivors continue to experience pain.

The best strategy to address pain depends on understanding the pain factors:

- Type and cause: is the pain a result of injury to tissues (skin, organs, muscle, bones, etc.) ("nociceptive"), or is it caused by injury to nerves ("neuropathic")?
- Intensity (rated on a 10-point scale, with 10 being the most severe)
- What makes it worse or better?
- How is it affecting you physically and emotionally?
- Current and past pain therapies
- Family and caregiver support
- Goals and expectations of pain management

Pain severity, duration, and location determine the appropriate pharmaceutical therapy:

- **Mild pain** (rating 1–3): Start with non-opioid analgesics (NSAIDs, acetaminophen). Adjuvant analgesics (antidepressants, anticonvulsants, topical agents, corticosteroids) can enhance effects.

- **Moderate pain** (rating 4–7): Non-opioid and adjuvant analgesics, with short-acting opioids as needed.
- **Severe pain** (rating 8–10): Short-acting opioid medications. Long-acting or extended-release opioids may be prescribed for chronic persistent pain (often lasting 12 or more hours each day) that is managed with short-acting opioids.
- **Breakthrough pain** while taking a long-acting opioid: Short-acting, rapid onset "rescue dose" opioids. Transmucosal (under the tongue or inside the cheek) fentanyl products are FDA-approved as breakthrough medication.

With any opioid prescription, your provider will counsel you on possible adverse effects.

Chemotherapy-induced peripheral neuropathy (CIPN) is common, typically develops in the first two months of treatment, and can worsen as treatment progresses. Fortunately, symptoms improve or resolve in most people within three to six months of completing treatment.

Unfortunately, there's no drug targeted specifically at CIPN. Because pharmaceutical therapies are not very effective for CIPN, integrative oncologists tend to combine complementary approaches. Talk with your care team about these options (listed alphabetically) and recommended practitioners.

Acupuncture can help restore nerve function in people with CIPN. Studies have shown that acupuncture increases blood flow in the limbs, aiding in oxygenation and nutrient delivery to the affected tissues and nerves. Choose an acupuncturist with experience in working with people who have cancer.

Biofeedback can be a useful therapy for CIPN. Biofeedback uses a special machine to help teach you to voluntarily control certain body functions such as heartbeat, blood pressure, and muscle tension, which can help control pain.

Cannabinoids. Pharmaceutical studies have found that the use of a full-spectrum CBD–THC (1:1 ratio) cannabis extract can reduce neuropathic pain symptoms by 30%, and higher in those with severe chronic pain of any type. (See p. 80)

Capsaicin patch. High-concentration 8-percent capsaicin patches (capsaicin is the spicy compound in chili peppers), which require a prescription, have been found to help in the management of neuropathic symptoms (not specifically CIPN). The capsaicin patch is normally applied with local anesthetic, left in place for 60 minutes and then removed. The effect lasts about 12 weeks. Significantly lower-dosed capsaicin patches and creams are available over the counter; while they may not be quite as effective, studies show that they, too, can help reduce pain.

Cognitive Behavioral Therapy (CBT) is based on the concept that thoughts are an important factor in how the mind and body process physical sensations, such as CIPN. Therapists and psychologists who practice CBT teach new ways to think about these sensations which help to relieve discomfort. CBT has proved helpful for people with pain syndromes (not specifically CIPN) during and after cancer treatment.

Cryotherapy. Wearing cold gloves and slippers decreases the blood flow to the tissues, thereby diminishing the amount of toxic chemotherapy drugs reaching the nerves in your extremities. (Similar to the cold cap method described on p. 47.)

Exercise. In one study, a six-week, home-based, moderate-intensity exercise program (walking and resistance exercise) significantly reduced CIPN symptoms in people receiving chemotherapy compared to those in a control group.

Guided imagery is a form of meditation that directs your imagination through verbal suggestion. Guided imagery has been reported to be helpful for patients with pain syndromes during and after cancer treatment. (See link to the guided imagery recordings we recommend on p. 60)

Hypnosis and self-hypnosis, a technique that combines guided imagery and meditation, may help people with managing pain syndromes during and after cancer treatment, particularly cancer treatment-related pain in children. You can teach yourself this technique with training from a medical hypnosis specialist (individually or in a group session), or through books, CDs, or DVDs. (See links to hypnosis resources on p. 60)

Lidocaine. Applying a daily 5% lidocaine patch over the affected skin can reduce CIPN pain.

Low Level Light Therapy (LLLT), Cold Laser Therapy, and Infrared Light Emitting Diode (LED) Therapy produce a low-energy light that penetrates up to an inch below the skin surface. Studies have shown that these therapies not only reduce pain but also speed up the body's natural healing mechanisms.

Massage may facilitate the healing of nerves by improving blood circulation to the affected tissues. Massage also increases the production of endorphins, the body's own pain-killing compounds.

Meditation focuses your awareness on an activity (your breath, relaxing music) and away from the distractions of your surroundings or the thoughts racing around in your head. Research indicates that meditation can reduce CIPN symptoms. (See p. 248)

Menthol. Applying topical 1% menthol cream twice daily to the affected skin has been shown to reduce CIPN symptoms in up to 81% of patients.

Occupational therapy. Occupational therapy can help you cope with CIPN's impact on various aspects of your life. It helps improve sensory and motor skills, teaches self-care activities and safety awareness, and provides techniques for maintaining mobility, stability, and range of motion with your hands and fingers.

Physical therapy. Physical therapy aims to help improve quality of life by increasing range of motion, strength, flexibility, balance, and avoiding pain-causing activities or movements. A physical therapist with experience in CIPN can formulate a personalized treatment plan for you that may include a variety of approaches: soft tissue techniques, padding over painful skin areas, heat therapies, electrical stimulation (such as TENS, below), ultrasound, vibrational platforms, LED or LLLT therapies, balance systems, and therapeutic exercise.

Scrambler therapy (ST) works by noninvasively electrically stimulating a specific type of pain sensory nerve, called C fibers.

Transcutaneous Electrical Nerve Stimulation (TENS) stimulates the A-beta pain nerve fibers using surface electrodes to decrease the excitability of these neurons.

Yoga has been found to provide reduction in physical and psychological CIPN symptoms. (See p. 245)

Over to You: Pain and Neuropathy Action Plan

- There are many different types of pain and, accordingly, many potential treatments. If the first one doesn't work, don't despair—try a different approach.
- In addition to the conventional medical pain treatments your doctors may offer you, there are many non-pharmaceutical interventions you can try; work through the list above to find one or several that sound good to you. Give them time—sometimes you have to make several attempts before you get the hang of, say, meditation or hypnotherapy.
- Get emotional support from professionals and loved ones; you shouldn't struggle alone.

15. Physical Limitations

Physical impairment caused by cancer treatment can hamper your recovery and shorten your life unnecessarily. Interventions can increase your strength, endurance, flexibility, and quality of life; reduce pain; and lower your risk of dying from non-cancer causes. Studies have shown that diet and exercise programs can reduce the post-treatment decline in physical function in the majority of participants.

Before you start any exercise routine, select a physical therapist and personal trainer educated and experienced in working with cancer survivors. The American College of Sports Medicine (acsm.org) offers a database of Certified Cancer Exercise Trainers, a program co-sponsored by the American Cancer Society (acsm.org/get-stay-certified/get-certified/specialization/cet).

Build muscle mass. While much attention has been focused on the anticancer effects of being physically active (i.e., getting 150 minutes per week of moderate intensity physical activity, etc.), one of the most important physiological changes you can make to your body is to focus on building muscle mass.

Studies indicate that the greater your muscle mass, the lower your risk of dying from the most common causes of death in U.S. adults: heart disease, diabetes, dementia, and cancer.

The reasons for this are complex, but are due in large part to the following:

- Muscle tissue consumes more energy (glucose, amino acids, fatty acids, and ketones) than any other tissue type in the body, increasing the body's basal metabolic rate and thus the calories burned.
- Muscle tissues release numerous immune-stimulating, anticancer, and anti-inflammatory proteins (myokines).
- The greater a person's muscle mass, the greater their exercise tolerance and ability to perform activities of daily living. Debility necessarily leads to diminished overall health and quality of life.

- As a person's muscle mass increases, they have a larger storage capacity for dietary carbohydrates/glucose. This in turn reduces insulin resistance.
- Building muscle strength is one of the most important physiological factors associated with increasing bone density, and preventing osteopenia/osteoporosis. Research suggests that the more muscle mass people have, the more effective immunotherapy drugs work on their cancer.

Approach muscle building (see p. 194) like any other must-do treatment. If you're healthy enough to exercise, include muscle building exercises in your weekly routine. You don't need to exercise every day or spend hours lifting weights at a gym; you can do muscle-building exercises at home using your body weight, resistance bands, or weights.

Before you start a new exercise routine, meet with a physical therapist who is experienced in working with people with cancer to determine any physical limitations you might have. Next, start your exercise program with a fitness trainer who is experienced in working with cancer patients/survivors. (Strength training is not recommended for people who are extremely ill; for instance, if they have cachexia, sepsis, organ failure, bowel obstruction, acute injuries, etc.).

Look into HIIT. While muscle building is essential to health, it's also important to keep your cardiovascular system in good shape. If you don't have a lot of time for cardio workouts, we recommend you look into high-intensity interval training (HIIT), a cardiovascular exercise strategy alternating short periods of intense exercise with less intense recovery periods, until too exhausted to continue.

Most HIIT workouts take less than 30 minutes, and some are much shorter than that. Studies show positive anticancer effects after just one session of HIIT. Other studies report that cancer survivors who do HIIT have significant improvements in their quality of life and multiple physiologic variables after only a few months. Ask your trainer for a HIIT routine that meets your needs and limitations.

Over to You: Physical Limitations Action Plan

- Don't assume that physical impairments resulting from your cancer treatment are irreversible; discuss them with your doctor and make a plan to address them
- Exercise is one of the most effective ways to counter physical impairments from cancer treatment
- Prioritize muscle building
- Work with a physical therapist and/or fitness instructor who specializes in working with cancer patients/survivors
- Be gentle with yourself; Rome was not built in a day

16. Radiation Dermatitis

Many people undergoing radiation treatments develop a skin reaction called radiation dermatitis (RD), characterized by redness, itchiness, peeling, dryness, sensitivity, blistering, ulceration, and pain. Up to 85% of people treated with radiation develop moderate to severe skin reactions.

RD can develop within days to weeks after starting treatment and typically evolves as the treatment progresses. In the majority of cases, RD will start to resolve within a few days after the completion of treatment, but it can take four to eight weeks to fully recover.

Many topical products can reduce the severity of RD. Apply these creams, lotions, oils, or products with these ingredients to radiated skin two to four times per day until skin reactions have mostly resolved:

- Calendula (Miaderm, Boiron)
- Epigallocatechin-3-gallate (EGCG), a green tea extract

- B-sitosterol, an ingredient of beeswax and sesame oil (marketed as moist exposed burn ointment, "MEBO")
- Boswellia, a frankincense extract
- Curcumin, a turmeric extract
- Hyaluronic acid
- Corticosteroids
- Mepitel® film (breathable film applied preventively over radiated skin area)
- Atorvastatin
- Trolamine
- Silver sulfadiazine (SSD)
- Silver nylon dressing, a nonadherent dressing
- Cooling hydrogel dressing

Homemade skin soother. The following supplements are available as capsules. Break capsules and empty into a small spray bottle with 8–12 oz of filtered water.

- Boswellia, 350 mg
- Curcumin, 500 mg
- Green tea, 250 mg

Spray on radiation-damaged skin three to four times daily; let air dry. Apply spray at least 15–30 minutes apart from applying other topical products. Keep the mixture in a cool and dark location. Discard and make a new batch after 24 hours. Use this in combination with any of the above-mentioned topic creams, lotions, or oils.

Over to You: Radiation Dermatitis Action Plan

- Ask your doctor which of the above-listed topical treatments is appropriate for you; try a few until you find one that works for you
- Make a bottle of homemade herbal skin soother
- Eat an anti-inflammatory diet that includes fatty fish, plenty of vegetables and fruits (especially those containing a flavonoid called quercetin

that's found in onions, apples, berries, broccoli, spinach), and probiotic foods (see p. 174 for more information about anti-inflammatory foods)

17. Radiation Fibrosis

Radiation therapy sometimes causes tissue fibrosis, an accumulation of fibrous tissue, often in the breast, head, neck, arms, and legs. Areas of fibrosis feel rubbery, firm, or hard to the touch.

Ask about PTX/vitamin E therapy. According to research, the conventional drug pentoxifylline (PTX) and vitamin E may help. In one study, patients who took a regimen of vitamin E and PTX, starting immediately after completing breast radiation and continuing for six months, had 50% less fibrosis than those who did not. Ask your radiation oncologist whether you're a good candidate for PTX/vitamin E therapy. If so, start the treatment before starting radiation therapy, but especially after completing it.

Get a massage. Therapeutic massage has also been shown to relieve radiation-induced skin fibrosis. Not every massage therapist can do this type of massage, so work with a physical therapist or certified lymphedema therapist who has experience in massaging radiated tissues.

Investigate Hyperbaric Oxygen Therapy (HBOT). Hyperbaric oxygen therapy—breathing 100% oxygen while inside a pressurized chamber—may be a very effective treatment for radiation-damaged tissues, even damage caused by prior (rather than current) radiation treatment.

Hundreds of studies demonstrate that a course (20–40 "dives") of HBOT can regrow bone and tissue in damaged areas of the body. That's because tissue oxygenation encourages new blood vessels to grow, which carry extra blood and nutrients to the damaged tissues. HBOT can also increase the ability of white blood cells to kill bacteria and prevent infection, and reduce swelling, pressure, and pain.

In addition to fibrosis, HBOT also helps with other radiation side effects, such as:

- decreased range of motion
- chronic pain
- chronic bladder or rectal inflammation, bleeding, urgency or frequency in urination or bowel movements
- necrosis or exposed bone
- neuropathy
- delayed wound healing

Caution: While HBOT data is promising, there are significantly higher risks of side effects, so it remains a non-standard therapy. Ask your radiation oncologist if a referral to an HBOT evaluation center might be helpful in your situation.

Over to You: Fibrosis Action Plan

- Book a therapeutic massage
- Talk to your doctor about PTX/vitamin E therapy
- Ask your doctor whether hyperbaric oxygen treatment may be appropriate for you

18. Skin and Nail Damage

Skin reactions to drug therapies are very common and include rashes, dryness, sensitivity, acne-like pimples, and redness or darkening.

Wash gently. When showering or bathing, minimize the use of soap; limit it to your armpits, groin, hands, and feet rather than using it over your whole body. Use mild soap and lukewarm water. Take showers or short, cool baths, rather than long, hot baths.

Moisturize. Apply a moisturizing cream or lotion to your hands, feet, and any dry areas at least once per day. Apply immediately after your shower or bath while your skin is still moist.

Avoid additives. Use fragrance-free and dye-free soaps, shampoos, detergents, lotions, creams, and oils. We like soaps and lotions made from natural substances like olive oil, beeswax, lanolin, etc. You can find these at health food stores, or even make them yourself. (Conner makes body butter, face scrub, and lip balm using Stephanie Tourles' 2007 book, *Organic Body Care Recipes: 175 Homemade Herbal Formulas for Glowing Skin & a Vibrant Self.)*

Wear loose clothes. To minimize friction and irritation to skin, wear loose-fitting clothing and undergarments over affected areas.

Use sun protection. Even when it's cloudy, apply broad spectrum UVA/UVB sunscreen (SPF 50+) before going outside. Reapply every 60–90 minutes while in the sun (or right after you get out of the pool or ocean). Wear sun-protective clothing.

Soothe nails with Polybalm. Most chemotherapy drugs can cause inflammation in the nail bed, leading to ridges, discoloration, cracking, pain from bleeding under the nails, or complete nail loss. In a randomized study, the application of a plant-based nail balm, Polybalm, markedly reduced damage from chemotherapy. It's not a quick fix remedy; benefits will only be seen after several weeks' use as nails grow.

Skip the gel. Do not get "gel nail" manicures. These require UV light exposure to harden the polish and can cause nail loss or skin rashes.

Over to You: Skin and Nail Care Action Plan

- Minimize the use of soap on affected areas; keep showers or baths short and cool
- Use natural, fragrance-free body care products
- Use Polybalm on damaged nails

19. Sleep Problems

Many people nowadays struggle with sleep, but people undergoing cancer treatment tend to be particularly afflicted. Sleep disturbances, including sleeping too much, insomnia, or disrupted sleep, affect 30–75% of people with cancer.

We have a more detailed section on sleep on p. 213, but here are just a few suggestions that can make a real difference.

Have a sleep schedule. Going to bed and getting up around the same time each day helps to regulate your body clock (circadian rhythm) and can improve sleep. Since most people do best when they sleep 7–8 hours a night, we recommend going to bed no later than 10 pm and getting up at around 6 am, give or take half an hour.

Limit caffeine, sugar, and alcohol. Caffeine, a potent stimulant found in coffee, black tea, maté, cocoa/chocolate, and some sodas and medications, can disrupt sleep. It has a half-life of six hours, which means that if you drink a cup of coffee at 2 pm, half the caffeine in it will still be circulating at 8 pm. Three 8-oz cups of coffee (250 mg of caffeine) per day is considered a moderate amount of caffeine, but in some people, even this amount of caffeine can disrupt sleep. Experiment with reducing your caffeine intake or try cutting it out altogether. There are many delicious caffeine-free drinks available, including decaffeinated coffee that tastes just like the real thing.

Sugar and refined carbohydrates can disrupt sleep by causing blood-glucose fluctuations; a high-carb meal eaten before bedtime can cause a spike, followed by a slump, in blood glucose. If this happens while you're sleeping, your body will produce stress hormones like adrenaline or cortisol to raise your glucose level, which will cause you to wake up—sometimes feeling sweaty or shaky.

Alcohol, meanwhile, is a sleep fragmenter; while it may make us feel nicely drowsy right after ingesting it, it can disrupt our sleep cycles later in the night, particularly blocking REM sleep, or dream sleep, which is critical for mental health.

See daylight early in the day. Exposing yourself to direct daylight soon after waking also helps to regulate your circadian rhythm. If you're up to it, go for a walk soon after rising; if not, sit on your balcony or patio to sip your tea or coffee. Or, in the winter, sit in front of a light box as soon as you get up (see p. 33).

Avoid bright light at night. Being exposed to artificial light at night blocks the production of melatonin, our body's sleep hormone (which also has cancer-protective and antioxidant properties), by up to 80%. Try to keep lights dim in the evening, minimize time spent looking at backlit screens (TV, computers, tablets, and smartphones). For extra protection, install blue-light blocking filters on your devices and wear blue-light blocking glasses at night.

4-7-8 Breath. This breathing technique is a powerful and effective relaxation method that you can do anywhere, at any time. It's a highly effective antidote to stress and insomnia—we usually recommend it to people who have trouble going (back) to sleep. Adapted from a yoga breathing practice (pranayama), it was popularized by Andrew Weil, M.D., Director of the Arizona Center for Integrative Medicine at the University of Arizona.

1. **Get into a comfortable position.** Try either a seated position, with hands on lap, or lie down.
2. **Press the tip of your tongue** on the ridge of tissue just behind your top front teeth. Keep it there throughout the breathing cycles.
3. **Breathe in deeply** *through your nose* for **4** seconds.
4. **Hold your breath** for **7** seconds.
5. **Breathe out slowly** *through your mouth* for **8** seconds. As you exhale, you will be blowing the air around your tongue, which remains pressed on the ridge of tissue behind your front teeth.
6. **Repeat steps 3–5** for three or more breathing cycles.

Do this at least three or four times a day. You can gradually increase the number of cycles over the next few weeks, but don't do more than 10 cycles in a row. It's normal to feel lightheaded at first, but this will pass as you get more comfortable and as your body adjusts to the technique.

Over to You: Better Sleep Action Plan

1. Plan a sleep schedule; set reminders on your phone to help you stick to it
2. Spend time outdoors, especially during the first half of the day
3. Reduce light at night
4. Cut caffeine, sugar, and alcohol
5. Practice breathing exercises

20. Unintended Weight Loss

Cancer treatments may reduce your appetite, change the way food tastes or smells, or make you too tired to prepare meals. Treatment-related side effects, such as problems with chewing and swallowing, nausea, or vomiting, can also put you off your food and can lead to weight loss.

Chapter 6 discusses how to deal with involuntary weight loss, starting on p. 205.

Start with these tips:

- **Plan ahead.** Buy a cookbook or two, including Conner's *Zest for Life: The Mediterranean Anticancer Diet* and the recipe books for people with cancer and survivors published by *Optimising Nutrition* (app.optimisingnutrition.com/cancer-recipe-books) that contain recipes for healthy, tasty meals. Cook (or ask someone else to cook) some nutritious meals and freeze them. Ask a friend to line up other friends to prepare nutritious meals for you, once your treatments start.

- **Book a consultation** with a nutrition professional to design a meal plan calculated to help you maintain your weight.
- **Talk to your care team** as soon as any eating difficulties arise, either before or during treatment. Don't wait until you feel weak and have lost more than three or four lbs.

Gain weight healthfully. Cancer itself can increase some people's calorie requirements, especially those with advanced cancers. When you're underweight, you need to eat more than you would to simply maintain your weight.

As a rule of thumb, you should take in an extra 300–500 calories a day to gain weight slowly and steadily (about half to one pound per week).Increase calorie intake gradually to avoid indigestion and overwhelm. Track your food intake on a food journaling app, such as Cronometer.

Many of our clients tell us: "My doctor said I should eat cookies and ice cream to gain weight"; others are told to drink commercial meal replacement drinks. Sorry—we disagree. You need nutritious calories, not empty ones.

Of course, the occasional cookie, scoop of ice cream, or protein shake is fine. But most brands of processed treats and meal replacement drinks are low in nutrients and packed with sugar and low-quality proteins and fats. So while they supply calories, they also provide compounds that may fuel the growth of your cancer, which is the last thing you want.

If you are underweight, the best way to increase calorie intake is to incorporate healthy fats into your diet. That's because fat contains more than twice as many calories as proteins or carbohydrates. While protein will help you build muscle mass (as long as you are doing resistance exercise) and body weight, ratcheting up the amount of fat calories in your diet can help you more quickly regain weight.

Easy ways to eat nutritious calories. To eat more calories, increase your fat intake:

- Eat a tablespoon of unsweetened almond or coconut butter
- Add a hunk of cheese to your meal
- Instead of water, drink a glass of high-fat nut milk (Conner's website, modernmediterranean.com, features recipes for homemade nut and seed milks) organic sheep, goat, or cow's milk, or make a smoothie with full-fat coconut milk
- Add a homemade protein shake to your breakfast or as an extra meal; use plant-based protein powders
- Make sugar-free cocoa or eggnog using high-fat nut milk or coconut milk
- Add heavy cream or nut milk to coffee or tea
- Drink a "bullet-proof" coffee blended with organic coconut oil and ghee or butter
- Eat an avocado
- Eat a bowl of berries covered with coconut cream (flavor this with a little stevia and vanilla extract, if you like)
- Use extra virgin olive oil for salad dressings; it's also fine to cook with at temperatures below 400°F; snack on olives
- Use high-quality avocado oil for cooking or salad dressings; use 100% avocado-oil mayonnaise; top salads, chilis or omelets with diced avocado
- Use coconut oil and ghee (clarified butter) for cooking, baking and roasting
- Eat nuts (raw and unsalted), nut butters, and nut oils
- Consume seeds (chia, flax, hemp, sunflower, pumpkin)—add these to smoothies, stir them into coconut porridge or sprinkle them over salads and soups
- Use almond oil, walnut oil, hazelnut oil, macadamia oil, and MCT oil (a flavorless, odorless coconut oil that's easy to absorb) for salad dressings and in smoothies
- Savor Mediterranean dips and herb emulsions that contain olive oil, like pesto, salsa verde, hummus, roasted eggplant dip (baba ganoush) or tzatziki

- Drink high-fat plant milks such as hemp, hazelnut, pumpkin-seed or flax milk
- Enjoy dark chocolate, 75% cocoa content or higher
- Stir a few tablespoons of a healthy oil into hot drinks, grains, soups, and bean dishes
- Eat oily fish
- Add healthy oils or nut butters to smoothies, oatmeal or coconut porridge, mashed potatoes, salad dressings, and cooked or raw vegetables

And avoid:

- Industrially processed fats, such as soybean, canola, corn, sunflower, and safflower oils
- Trans fats, found in margarines, hydrogenated oils, and processed and fried foods

Eat protein for muscle mass and strength. You need protein (see p. 96) to build muscle tissue and cells throughout the body—vitally important if cancer treatment causes lost weight and muscle mass (cachexia, p. 205).

For most adults, we recommend that you consume at least 0.5–1.0 grams of protein per pound of ideal body weight each day (estimate your ideal body weight using this calculator: calculator.net/ideal-weight-calculator.html. This calculator doesn't take body shape into account; we merely use it here to help you calculate your estimated protein requirement.) Foods that provide high-quality protein include:

- Fish and seafood
- Meat
- Eggs
- Yogurt
- Protein powder

Eat carbs for energy. Minimally refined carbohydrates are a great source of minerals, vitamins, and fiber. They gently increase blood glucose (which provides energy) and insulin (which encourages fat storage and muscle synthesis).

Focus on nutritious carbs, such as:

- Vegetables

- Fruits
- Legumes (beans, chickpeas, lentils, etc., preferably soaked and cooked from scratch)

Eat low-glycemic carbs (see p. 108) at every meal, but don't overdo high-fiber vegetables, which can fill you up without providing many calories.

Avoid refined, processed carbs (candy and desserts, pasta, white rice, soda, beer), which lack nutrients and can upset your blood sugar balance and fuel inflammation.

Again, we want to emphasize that it's important to limit your carbohydrate intake to 50–100 "net" carbs per day to reduce the swings in blood sugar and insulin that could fuel your cancer. (More on carbs on p. 104)

Digest and absorb well. Usually, we recommend eating no more than three meals a day, but when you're trying to gain weight—especially when your appetite is low—five or six small meals a day may be helpful. Chew your food thoroughly and relax when you're eating. This helps your body break down and absorb nutrients from the foods you eat.

If you can't chew or swallow solid food, drink your meals. Milkshakes, smoothies, vegetable juices, smooth soups, and broths—notably protein-rich bone broth—can provide easy-to-digest nutrients. Consult a nutritionist or dietitian for more ideas.

Chemotherapy may deplete digestive enzymes and healthy bacteria needed to digest food and absorb its nutrients. Digestive supplements can help; ask your doctor or nutritionist.

Use weights. Just as with weight loss, weight gain relies on physical activity. Build lean muscle mass through weight training. Begin lightly and increase weights gradually. When you start to recover strength, increase workout intensity gradually and add a little cardio training (walking, cycling, treadmill). None of this should be strenuous; ask a fitness trainer or physical therapist to design an exercise program that's appropriate for you.

Over to You: Weight Gain Action Plan

- Eat healthy fats
- Eat high-quality protein
- Eat minimally processed carbs
- Eat frequent, small meals and chew your food thoroughly
- Talk to a nutritionist or dietitian about supplements to optimize digestion and gut health
- Start a gentle weight-training routine

Cannabis 101

Though long associated with hippie stoners and rebellious teenagers, cannabis (also known as marijuana, weed, dope, and more) is increasingly seen as an effective tool in managing cancer-related symptoms.

Cannabinoids, found in the cannabis plant, are a class of chemicals that alter neurotransmitter release in the brain—and offer anticancer benefits. In the US, as of May 2021, 36 states and the District of Columbia permit doctor-prescribed cannabis for certain medical conditions. A growing number of states permit it recreationally.

In a recent survey of cancer patients at Seattle Cancer Care Alliance, in Washington, where medical and recreational cannabis is legal, 75% of active cannabis users were taking it for cancer-related symptoms (pain, nausea, appetite, stress, depression, insomnia). The survey also found that 74% of people wanted to learn about cannabis from their healthcare providers, but were unable to glean enough information from them.

A 2018 national survey of oncologists found that 80% had discussions about medical marijuana with patients. But less than 30% of the surveyed oncologists felt knowledgeable enough about medical marijuana to make recommendations, even though:

- 67% of oncologists believed medical marijuana to be helpful for alleviating pain when used together with standard therapies
- Most believed that it poses a lower risk than opioids for overdose death (75%) and addiction (52%)
- 65% viewed it as equally or more effective than standard treatments for poor appetite and extreme weight loss

Unfortunately, decades of legal prohibition have attached a stigma to this botanical compound—including in medical circles.

What is cannabis? Cannabis is a plant with two species:

- Hemp: legal because it contains no more than 0.3% of the psychoactive compound THC
- Marijuana: illegal in many states because it contains more than 0.3% THC.

The cannabis plant contains over 400 chemical compounds, including more than 60 cannabinoids, the molecules that exert most of the pharmacological activity.

The main psychoactive compound is delta-9-THC, simply called THC. In 1986, the FDA approved a synthetic delta-9-THC for treating chemotherapy-associated nausea and vomiting. In 1992, it was approved for poor appetite and weight loss in people with HIV.

Cannabis's second most prevalent active compound is cannabidiol (CBD). Most CBD is derived from hemp. Unlike THC, CBD does not generate a "high." In fact, CBD inhibits the psychoactive effects of THC.

Currently, most people use hemp-derived CBD, legally purchased through websites or CBD retailers. CBD is commonly used to address anxiety, insomnia, and chronic pain conditions, although there is a lack of high-quality clinical studies to support these indications.

Cannabinoids in the body. Perhaps the most exciting area of cannabinoid research involves the discovery of the human body's endocannabinoid system. Incredibly, this system makes cannabis-like chemicals that interact with and stimulate cannabinoid receptors in cells. CBD directly interacts with the body's opioid, dopamine, and serotonin receptors, which likely explains its broad effects.

Studies continue to uncover the numerous functions of the human endocannabinoid system. Anticancer implications include:

- Anti-inflammatory activity
- Antioxidant activity
- Inhibiting tumor cell growth and promoting cancer cells' self-destruction
- Inhibiting blood vessel growth to tumors
- Antiviral activity
- Neuroprotective effects
- Immune system modulation

Dr. Lawenda often recommends a trial of cannabis or cannabinoid extract as an optional therapy to help people undergoing cancer treatment better manage:

- Nausea
- Diminished appetite (and associated weight loss)
- Pain
- Sleeping difficulties
- Anxiety, stress, and depression

In many cases, cannabinoids can address all five symptoms and can be significantly less expensive than many pharmaceuticals, with fewer side effects. Many people report that using cannabinoids enables them to decrease use of drugs for pain, anxiety, sleeping problems, and nausea.

Combining pharmaceuticals with cannabinoids is usually safe *but should only be done after getting approval from your oncology healthcare providers*. Dangerous interactions are theoretically possible, so it's essential to check first.

Cannabinoid delivery systems:

- Edibles: oils, baked products, butters, teas, gum, beer, candies
- Sublinguals (under the tongue): oils, liquid sprays, tinctures

- Inhalation: smoking or vaporizing
- Topicals: creams, oils, lotions, patches
- Suppositories: rectal or vaginal

Sublingual (tinctures, oils) and inhalational (smoking or vaporizing) routes offer the fastest onset (1–15 minutes) and shortest duration of effects (0.5–2 hours).

Edibles, suppositories, and topicals offer the slowest onset (0.5–2 hours) and longest duration of effects (4–10 hours or longer).

Unfortunately, most CBD-rich hemp tinctures have a very low bioavailability. A new type of product formulation, called nanoencapsulation, significantly increases CBD bioavailability; that means you can absorb twenty times more CBD per drop of tincture than you would otherwise. Nanoencapsulated tinctures can be added to drinks and maintain their high bioavailability.

Look for "full spectrum" products, which contain a wide range of cannabinoids and other organic compounds. The combination often leads to synergistic ("entourage") effects, which may improve the desired effectiveness of the cannabinoid product. Read labels and choose products made with either ethanol alcohol or supercritical CO_2 extraction.

What's the right dose? It takes trial and error to know how much of any cannabinoid product is right for each person and condition. Start with the smallest dose and slowly increase the amount until you reach the desired effect or until you experience undesirable side effects. Cannabis can have a biphasic effect, where lower doses cause one effect and higher doses cause the opposite effect. For example:

- Low dose (energizing) vs. high dose (sedating)
- Low dose (superior pain reduction) vs. high dose (less pain reduction)
- Low dose (reduced anxiety or stress) vs. high dose (increased anxiety and paranoia)

Cannabis for pain. When using cannabis to address chronic pain, choose a long-acting administration method.

Edibles often last 4–10 hours and provide a steady state of cannabinoids to help alleviate pain.

Since breakthrough pain, nausea, and other acute symptoms occur quickly but less frequently, sublingual and vaporized CBD products provide much quicker relief and last approximately 30 minutes to two hours.

In most cases, cancer patients seem to respond best with a CBD-to-THC ratio of 1:1. Many people feel this is too potent to start; to build up tolerance, start with a 4:1 ratio for two weeks, then a 2:1 ratio for two weeks, and then a 1:1 ratio.

Keep both an edible (long-acting and slow onset) product and a sublingual tincture or vape (short-acting and rapid onset) product handy to manage chronic side effects, such as pain. *Again, get approval from your oncologist first.*

Smoke or vape? Burning herbs and tobacco produces toxins and carcinogens, and filters and water pipes (bongs, hookahs) remove only a fraction of these dangerous molecules. An electric vaporizer, which heats plant material to a temperature that produces vapor without combustion, is a safer inhalational option.

Beware: Some vaporizers use liquid cannabis or solid resin concentrates—but hospitals across the U.S. have reported thousands of cases of people who have developed lung injury or died after using these products. The FDA warns consumers to stop using THC vaping products. (This risk has not been seen with the use of dried cannabis vaporizers or when smoking cannabis.

Are cannabinoids safe? Research indicates that when used correctly, cannabinoids very safe—especially compared with many prescription drugs.

That said, cannabinoids are active drugs with potential risks and side effects. These may include rapid heartbeat, low blood pressure, muscle relaxation, bloodshot eyes, slowed digestion, dizziness, depression, hallucinations, and paranoia. Even CBD has potential side effects, including nausea, fatigue, and irritability.

THC-containing cannabis—but not CBD—may cause use dependence (feeling withdrawal symptoms when not taking it) or addiction (cannot stop using even though it interferes with life). In 2015, about four million people in the United States met the diagnostic criteria for a marijuana use disorder; 138,000 voluntarily sought treatment. If you think you're becoming addicted to cannabis, talk to your doctor about how to wean yourself off it.

Chapter 3

Eat to Beat Cancer

For many years, conventional doctors pooh-poohed the idea that diet and nutrition were important in cancer prevention and treatment. Don't blame them; most medical schools haven't taught their physicians about nutrition. Thankfully, the vital role of nutrition is now increasingly understood—not only as a way to reduce the risk of developing cancer but also during cancer treatment and beyond.

Nutritional Chemoprevention

Due to normal physiological processes, our bodies produce and carry microscopically small tumors every day of our lives. In many cases, our own defense systems (see chapter 4) nip these microtumors in the bud. But when those defenses are disturbed, tiny tumors can develop into life-threatening cancers.

"Nutritional chemoprevention" is a process through which a wide range of cancer-fighting nutrients, ingested several times a day, every day, can help protect you by creating an environment that is hostile to invasive tumors. These nutrients can help:

- Shield cells from free-radical damage
- Remove toxins from the body
- Reduce inflammation
- Prompt any precancerous cells to self-destruct

- Prevent any precancerous cells from progressing into malignant tumors

No single food possesses all the molecules needed to act on all the stages of cancer development, and there's no list of proven "anticancer" foods. But eating the broadest possible range of nutritious foods—especially plant foods—can create a multipronged attack on cancer cells that's not unlike the multidrug regimens that oncologists often prescribe.

Eat Like Your Ancestors

Ancestral diets around the world have a lot in common. They consist mostly of whole foods, locally produced and eaten close to their natural state. These diets are rich in plant foods packed with nutrients and fiber. And they use traditional food-preparation techniques, including soaking, sprouting, fermentation, drying, and slow cooking.

Unfortunately, the transition many of us have made from those traditional ancestral diets to refined and processed foods—a process known as "nutrition transition"—often leads to diseases prevalent in more "advanced" industrial societies: heart disease, obesity, type 2 diabetes, and cancer. In some recently developing countries, such as China, India, and Brazil, these diseases are on the rise and occurring in ever younger people.

The Mediterranean Diet

Because of its wide nutrient range, the Mediterranean diet—not a time-limited "diet," but a time-honored eating pattern—is probably the closest thing to an optimal diet to protect against cancer. (Other ancestral eating patterns may be similarly protective but haven't been studied in as much detail.)

Mediterranean Cancer Protection

Study after study of people who eat the Mediterranean diet points to cancer risk reduction, including:

- colorectal
- prostate
- breast (including triple-negative disease)
- endometrial
- gastric
- bladder
- cervical
- biliary tract
- pancreatic
- lung

Many Mediterranean foods are thought to mitigate cancer risk through various mechanisms, such as:

- their antioxidant and anti-inflammatory effects (for instance, vegetables, fruits, herbs, spices, and olive oil)
- reducing tumor cell growth (such as oily fish)
- their chemoprotective effects (for instance, olive oil) and insulin-sensitizing nutrients (polyunsaturated fatty acids in oily fish, olive oil, and seeds; anthocyanins from purple vegetables and fruits; resveratrol from grapes; and a compound in extra virgin olive oil called oleacein)

Scientists estimate that up to 25% of colorectal cancers, 15% of breast cancers, and 10% of prostate, pancreatic, and endometrial cancers could be prevented if people did nothing more than adopt a Mediterranean diet (see pubmed.ncbi.nlm.nih.gov/11008902).

The more elements of the Mediterranean diet that are incorporated, the greater the protection. A large-scale European study conducted over 12 years showed that when the Mediterranean diet was combined with other healthy lifestyle habits—for instance, taking regular exercise and not smoking—people were 65% more likely to outlive those who had none of these healthy habits, and were 60% less likely to die of cancer (see pubmed.ncbi.nlm.nih.gov/15383513).

The only controlled dietary investigation to date into the health effects of the Mediterranean diet yielded similar results. The Lyon Diet Heart Study indicated that eating a Mediterranean diet not only protected its 605 participants from cardiovascular disease but also from cancer. After four years, Mediterranean eaters were 61% less likely to develop cancer than members of the control group—this despite the fact that the control group members were eating the American Heart Association's so-called prudent diet! (See pubmed.ncbi.nlm.nih.gov/9625397.)

More recently, a 2015 study of more than 5,000 Italian women found that those who ate a Mediterranean diet had a 57% lower risk of endometrial (uterine) cancer than women who didn't. Moreover, they found that those who adhered mostly closely to this eating pattern had greater protection that those who only followed it loosely (see pubmed.ncbi.nlm.nih.gov/26010500).

Also in 2015, the *Journal of the American Medical Association* reported that postmenopausal, overweight Spanish women eating a traditional Mediterranean diet enhanced with extra virgin olive oil were 68% less likely to be diagnosed with breast cancer than those allocated to a lower-fat control diet (see pubmed.ncbi.nlm.nih.gov/26365989).

A carefully designed 2014 study reported that the Mediterranean dietary pattern was related to a 44% lower risk of breast cancer, especially triple-negative disease. Women with metabolic syndrome are more likely to have triple-negative breast cancer upon diagnosis than women without it. Systemic inflammation has been shown to increase the risk of metastasis in triple-negative breast cancer. The same study found that women eating a typical western diet high in processed meat, refined grains, high-fat dairy products, sweets, caloric drinks, and other convenience foods and sauces had a 56% higher risk of developing breast cancer than those who did not eat this way (see ncbi.nlm.nih.gov/pmc/articles/PMC4183855).

Even more recently, in 2017, a team of Dutch researchers studied a large group of postmenopausal women and found that eating a Mediterranean diet reduced their risk of estrogen receptor-negative breast cancer—which usually has a poorer prognosis than other types of breast cancer—by 40%, compared to those not eating this way (see pubmed.ncbi.nlm.nih.gov/28260236).

This is not to say that all Mediterranean-type foods reduce cancer risk. Alcohol—for instance, in wine or aperitifs popular in many Mediterranean countries—does not lower cancer risk. Neither do breads and pastas made with refined flour. If anything, they may increase your disease risk if you consume them frequently, and in large quantities.

For example, one Italian study reported that women in the highest third of intake of desserts (including cookies, brioche, cakes, pastry puffs, and ice cream) or sugars (including honey, jam, marmalade, and chocolate) had 1.2 times the risk of breast cancer as those in the lowest third (see ncbi.nlm.nih.gov/pmc/articles/PMC1283300). Another Italian study found that the risk of breast and colorectal cancers rose with increasing consumption of pastas and breads, particularly breads (see pubmed.ncbi.nlm.nih.gov/24155133).

Thus, when we recommend the Mediterranean diet, we're not referring to what Americans generally think of when they imagine Italian food: pasta, pizza, and gelato. We're talking about the sort of food that was widely eaten in the Mediterranean region before the advent of industrial food production: in-season vegetables and fruits, legumes, moderate amounts of intact grains, fermented dairy products, fresh eggs, moderate amounts of wild-caught fish and pastured meat, olive oil, nuts, seeds, herbs and spices. More on this in the coming sections.

Over to You: Mediterranean Action Plan

The list below describes the main features of the traditional Mediterranean diet and lifestyle. Check off the ones that are already part of your daily habits. Then, choose ones you don't yet practice and gradually integrate them into your daily life, one by one. (Sadly, many people in the Mediterranean basin no longer practice these behaviors, which explains a widespread increase in obesity and metabolic health problems in the region.)

- Lots of vegetables and some fruits (at least five servings a day, ideally more)
- Foods that are minimally processed (as close to their natural state as possible)
- Eating lots of *different* foods (variety)
- Healthy fats (like extra virgin olive oil, nuts, seeds, avocado, oily fish)
- When eating grains, consuming their intact, unprocessed form (such as farro, barley, brown rice, oat groats, quinoa)
- Low sugar intake
- Regular consumption of nuts, seeds, and legumes
- Rich in aromatic herbs and spices
- Oily fish two to three times a week
- Moderate amounts of eggs (ideally pastured)
- Moderate intake of dairy (ideally fermented; frequently sheep and goat)
- Moderate meat consumption (ideally pastured or grass-fed)
- Moderate alcohol intake, i.e., modest consumption of red wine with meals. (We don't recommend alcohol to anyone who is affected by cancer. More on this on p. 237)

- Conviviality, joy of eating, absence of food guilt
- Daily physical activity (can be gentle, like walking)
- Spending a lot of time outdoors and in nature (while avoiding the hot midday sun)
- Rest, relaxation, and adequate sleep (think siestas!)
- Close-knit communities, social interaction, and support

Macronutrient Balance

Food can be divided into two categories: macronutrients and micronutrients.

Macronutrients—protein, fat and carbohydrate—are those nutrients the body needs in large amounts; among others, they provide energy (calories). Micronutrients—minerals like calcium and zinc, and vitamins like B6 and C—are needed in much smaller amounts, but are no less important as they regulate thousands of bodily functions. Let's start by looking at macronutrients; we'll return to micronutrients later.

Given all the nutrition information out there, it's no wonder you may feel confused. Do carbohydrates feed cancer? What role does protein play? Does fat make you fat?

The truth is: carbohydrates, fats, and proteins—the three macronutrients—all play an important role in a healthy diet. However, some types of carbohydrate, fat, and protein are more nutritious than others, so it's important to prioritize the ones that provide the nutrition your body needs—and this can vary from one person to another.

Every meal or snack you eat should ideally provide some protein, some fat, and some carbohydrate. Macronutrient needs vary from one person to another depending on their weight, height, age, sex, activity level, and health status. An athlete may tolerate (and need) more carbohydrate than a sedentary individual; a person recovering from illness who has lost muscle mass may need more protein than a healthy person; and someone who wants to gain weight may do well to increase their fat intake. To find out your individual macronutrient requirements, ask a nutrition professional to calculate these for you.

Balance Your Meals

Many people eat most of their protein and fat at dinner, often prioritizing carbohydrates during the day (especially at breakfast). However, spreading all three macronutrients evenly across the day is the best way of ensuring satiety, balancing blood sugar levels, and providing your body with a steady supply of the nutrients it needs.

Most foods contain a combination of protein, fat, and carbohydrate, but in many foods one macronutrient dominates. For instance, fruits, vegetables, grains, and legumes are mostly made up of carbohydrate; nuts, seeds, and cheese are mostly fat; and chicken, non-oily fish, and reduced-fat yogurt are mostly protein.

Here are some examples of meals with well-balanced macronutrients:

Breakfast

- Spinach and onions (carbohydrate) braised in olive oil (fat) and scrambled with two eggs (protein, fat)
- Breakfast parfait: Plain, whole yogurt (protein, fat) layered with berries (carbohydrate) and homemade nut granola (fat, protein)
- Chia pudding: Chia seeds (protein, fat) with animal or plant milk (fat, protein), and berries (carbohydrate), and a few chopped nuts (fat, protein)

Lunch

- Greek salad: Tomatoes, cucumber, onion (carbohydrate) with feta cheese (fat, protein), olives (fat) and olive-oil dressing (fat)
- Leek, cabbage, and cannellini bean soup (carbohydrate) cooked in bone broth (protein), topped with a poached

egg (protein, fat), and sprinkled with Parmesan cheese (fat, protein)
- Toasted flaxseed bread (fat, protein) topped with chicken salad (protein, fat), accompanied by chopped cucumbers, grape tomatoes, and raw carrot (carbohydrate)

Dinner
- Broiled salmon (protein, fat) with roasted tomato and olive sauce (fat, carbohydrate) and butternut mash (carbohydrate)
- Chicken (protein) and chickpeas (carbohydrate, protein) braised with onions, tomatoes, and peppers (carbohydrate) in an herb-and-spice-rich Moroccan stew
- Stewing beef (protein, fat) slowly braised with onions, garlic, bell peppers, and black beans (carbohydrate) and drizzled with salsa verde (fat)

Snacks
- 1/2 cup plain, whole-milk Greek yogurt (protein, fat) topped with a chopped peach (carbohydrate)
- An apple (carbohydrate) with peanut butter, almond butter, or a handful of nuts (fat, protein)
- Roasted eggplant dip (fat, protein) on a gluten-free cracker (carbohydrate)

Eating all three macronutrients—proteins, fats, and carbohydrates—at every meal you eat is a great start, but there's more: they should ideally be of the highest quality you can find and afford. This means, where possible:
- Protein from animals reared under natural conditions—preferably organic, grass-fed, or wild-caught
- Unprocessed, natural fats as close to their natural state as possible
- Unrefined carbohydrates that are rich in vitamins, bioactive plant compounds, and fiber

More on food quality in the sections that follow.

Over to you: Macronutrient Balance Action Plan

- Starting with your next meal, look at your plate and ask yourself: "Where's my protein? Where's my fat? What's my carbohydrate?" If one macronutrient is missing, think of a way to add it to the meal. For instance, if you're eating mushroom risotto (carbs and fat), top it with grilled chicken or shrimp, or have some Greek yogurt as dessert.
- When planning meals, include a protein serving (for instance, meat, fish, seafood, eggs, dairy, tempeh), a carbohydrate serving (such as vegetables, fruits, beans, some sweet potato) and a fat serving (such as olive oil used for cooking, avocado, olive oil dressing, a sprinkling of pumpkin seeds).
- When you buy a packaged meal or snack, look for a healthy balance of protein, fat, and carbohydrate on the label.
- For a few days, track your meals on an app like Cronometer (cronometer.com) to see what your macronutrient distribution looks like. Ask a nutrition professional to help you determine the macronutrient balance that best suits you.

Food Journaling Pros and Cons

Let's face it: Most of us don't know much about nutrition. Not blaming anyone here, but since many of us don't learn about it at home or in school, most folks' dietary knowledge comes from articles we see on social media or the mainstream media (often poorly researched, biased, and commercially driven), TV advertising, and food packaging (ditto). Much of this information is contradictory and confusing.

And so most people compose meals based on what tastes good to them, what they tolerate, and what's fashionable or in line with their ethical values, rather than on the basis of nutritional balance. Unfortunately, even the most delicious vegan salad will be imbalanced if it's low in protein and fat; and a grain- and dairy-free paleo or keto breakfast won't nourish you optimally if it's laden with bacon and lacks fiber.

To help our clients better understand the foods they eat and to empower them to compose nutritionally balanced meals, we often recommend they use food trackers like Cronometer for a certain period of time.

Here's how they work: You enter the foods or meals you've eaten—or plan to eat (you can use trackers strategically to plan ahead)—and the tracker shows you how much protein, fat, carbohydrate, fiber, calcium, etc., you've consumed. This can be highly educational and motivating for anyone wishing to improve the nutritional quality of their diet.

On the downside, trackers can be time-consuming to use and often rely on poor-quality datasets that don't provide an accurate reflection of your diet. (To our knowledge, Cronometer has the most reliable data.) Moreover, they can lead to obsessive or restrictive eating behaviors, especially in people with a history of weight-loss dieting or disordered eating.

That's why we recommend that you don't use them long term. Trackers are based on fairly crude algorithms; they don't know your body as well as you do, so use them as a guide, but don't obey them blindly. They're like training wheels—you'll only need them until you can go it alone.

Limit tracking to a few days at a time—just long enough to learn, for example, how much protein is in a cup of chickpeas, what your best sources of omega-3 fatty acids are, and how to obtain the fiber you need.

Protein Power

The very origin of the word—from the Greek protos, meaning "first" or "most important"—reflects protein's top-shelf status in human nutrition. The body uses protein for hundreds of functions, including building cells; transporting oxygen and cholesterol; growing and repairing tissues such as muscle, bone, organs and ligaments; stabilizing blood sugar; and much more.

When you eat protein, your body breaks it down into subunits called amino acids that form new proteins. If you don't obtain all the essential amino acids from your diet, your body can't function properly.

To get the most from your protein, pay attention to:

- **Amino acid balance.** Animal proteins are described as "complete" because they contain the nine essential amino acids your body needs. Because most plant proteins are low in or lack an essential amino acid (making them "incomplete"), these can be harder to assimilate. Indeed, some nutrition experts estimate that ovo-lacto vegetarians should eat about 20% more protein than omnivores to meet their protein needs (see pubmed.ncbi.nlm.nih.gov/21167687). For vegans, who eat no animal protein at all, that percentage may be even higher. An additional drawback to getting most of your protein from legumes and grains is that these are high in carbohydrate, which, as you can read on pp. 105–117, may be problematic in the context of cancer.
- **Variety.** The best protein sources are fish, seafood, meat, dairy, and eggs. Legumes (including soy), nuts, seeds, whole grains, and vegetables also provide protein, but not nearly as much as animal-sourced foods, and not as absorbable. Try to vary animal and plant protein foods as much as possible to increase your chances of obtaining all the essential amino acids without getting too much of any one nutrient. For instance, some studies link egg yolks to certain types of cancer, like prostate or ovarian cancer; so, if you eat eggs frequently, consider reducing your egg intake by alternating them with other delicious protein foods.
- **Unprocessed.** Choose unprocessed protein (fresh meat, fish, seafood, eggs) rather than processed proteins

(luncheon meat, surimi, soy "bacon", soy protein isolates, highly processed protein powders, etc.).

- **Naturally produced.** Wherever possible, choose organic, grass-fed or pasture-reared animal protein. Prioritize wild-caught fish that are low in toxins (check seafoodwatch.org or ewg.org/seafood).
- **Gentle cooking.** Avoid high-temperature cooking, barbecuing, and flame-grilling; instead, braise or slow cook.

How Much Protein?

How much protein you need depends on your age, sex, height, weight, activity level, and overall health. If you're undergoing cancer treatment, or recovering from it, especially if you've lost weight or muscle mass, you'll need more protein than a healthy adult does. Dr. Lawenda recommends eating 5–10 grams of protein per 10 lbs of body weight, which is significantly more than the recommended daily allowance (for a healthy person) of 3.6 grams per 10 lbs of body weight. Meet with a nutrition professional to calculate your estimated protein requirement, or use Optimising Nutrition's free online Macro Calculator (optimisingnutrition.com/macro-calculator).

Many people with cancer struggle to meet protein needs through food alone. In this situation, take supplementary protein in the form of protein powders and drinks. Choose the least-processed protein supplement and make sure it contains no added sugar, flavorings, colorings, or other additives.

This advice also applies to commercial protein shakes and meal replacement drinks frequently recommended by oncologists. Most are chock full of sugar or artificial sweeteners, glycemic starches, unhealthy fats, flavorings, and other additives. For healthier options, we recommend:

- Orgain (orgain.com)
- OWYN (liveowyn.com)
- Ample (amplemeal.com)
- Maximum Vibrance (vibranthealth.com)

Gelatin and Collagen

Powdered gelatin and collagen offer an inexpensive and effective way to increase protein intake. People eating traditional diets get these compounds from bone broth and meat stews containing bones.

Gelatin is an interesting type of protein: it doesn't contain the amino acid tryptophan, and only small amounts of cysteine, methionine, and histidine—amino acids associated with many of the problems of aging and cancer. Gelatin does contain glycine, which has anti-inflammatory properties and a wide range of anticancer actions, including the inhibition of new blood vessel formation (angiogenesis).

You can purchase gelatin and collagen powders made from grass-fed beef and pork (e.g., at greatlakesgelatin.com). Mix 2 tablespoons with a little water, let it soften for three or four minutes, heat it briefly to dissolve, and then stir it into soups, stews, smoothies, or hot beverages such as chicken broth or hot cocoa. Or use it to make refreshing fruit gums: Dissolve the gelatin in juice, pour into ice-cube shapes, and chill until set.

Over to You: Protein Action Plan

- Ask a nutrition professional to help you calculate your protein requirement.
- Aim to eat a third of your protein requirement at each meal. Meal planning can make it easier to reach your targets at each meal.
- For the widest variety and best quality of amino acids, eat both animal and plant proteins.
- Track your meals on Cronometer to see whether you're reaching, under- or overshooting your targets. Don't obsess about getting it perfectly right; just try to more or less reach your targets on most days.

Focus on Fats

For the past 40 years dietary fat has been blamed for every imaginable disease, including heart attacks, weight gain, obesity, and even some cancers.

However, fats are essential to health. They provide energy. They nourish the brain and nervous system, protect vital organs, help regulate blood pressure and inflammation, contribute to healthy skin and eyes, assist hormone production, and build healthy cells. They act as carriers for important fat-soluble vitamins A, D, E, K and K2. Fats have no effect on blood-sugar levels; neither do they trigger the secretion of insulin. (More on this in the next section.)

Besides these biological roles, fats make meals more satisfying. They improve the mouthfeel and flavor of food, and help us feel satisfied for hours. This means we can go longer without feeling hungry, thus lessening our desire to reach for less nutritious snacks.

To be sure, some observational studies have linked fat—in particular, saturated fat—to increased cancer risk. This is an area of controversy and will likely remain so until much higher-quality prospective studies can be done to assess the true risk.

At this time, based on the available evidence, we do not believe the risk is significant. This is echoed by researchers at the Harvard School of Public Health in The Nutrition Source's online "Dietary Fat and Disease" article: "[I]n adults, the percentage of calories consumed from total fat appears to have no significant association with cancer risk, and there is currently no clear evidence linking any specific type of fat with cancer incidence."

As with protein, how much fat you need depends on various factors, including your age, sex, activity levels, the climate you live in, how cool or warm you keep your home, your general health, and more. Generally, some 35–40% of your calories can safely come from dietary fat—this percentage is typically consumed in the Mediterranean diet. In people eating low-carbohydrate or ketogenic diets (see p. 165), fat intake is sometimes as high as 75–80%.

As with protein, it's best to spread out your fat intake across the day. Most of the fats you eat should be "Mediterranean": olive oil, olives, nuts and seeds (and oils and butters made from these), avocado and oily fish (such as salmon, sardines, herring, mackerel, and anchovy). It's fine to eat some saturated fat too, ideally from traditionally reared animals: cheese and yogurt from grass-fed or organic dairy cows, sheep, and goats, pasture-fed beef and lamb, and eggs and meat from pastured chickens.

Optimize Your Omegas

While saturated and monounsaturated fats don't have a strong impact on cancer risk, some types of polyunsaturated fats may fuel cancer and inflammation, while other types weaken these processes.

Our bodies work best when essential fatty acids omega-6s and omega-3s are in a healthy balance. The ideal ratio for most humans is about two parts omega-6 to one part omega-3. Because omega-6s are abundant in processed foods, however, many people eat nearly 20 times more omega-6 fatty acids than omega-3 fatty acids.

This imbalance may cause health problems. An excess of omega-6 fatty acids can fuel inflammation, which encourages cancer cells to grow and spread, stimulates the production of tumor-promoting chemicals, and activates a gene that leads to uncontrolled cell replication and tumor growth.

Omega-3 fatty acids, on the other hand, have been shown to reduce inflammation, thin blood, and control cell growth. They can also enhance the effects of certain types of chemotherapy and radiation treatments, slow tumor growth, reverse tumor metastasis, and reduce the risk of wasting (cachexia) in cancer patients.

The best sources of omega-3 fatty acids are fatty fish (mackerel, salmon, herring, oysters, sardines, anchovies), flax seeds, chia seeds, walnuts, and green leafy vegetables. Meat, eggs, and dairy from grass-fed animals contain some omega-3 fats too.

Beneficial omega-6 fats are found in most nuts, seeds, and tofu. Less-healthy sources of omega-6 include industrially refined oils such as soybean, corn, sunflower, and cottonseed oils (which are frequently used to make processed and fast foods). The meat and milk from animals fattened with corn also tend to contain more omega-6 fatty acids. Diets high in refined omega-6s but low in omega-3s—typical of the standard American diet—are thought to drive inflammation and cancer growth.

Olive Oil

We recommend extra virgin olive oil for most culinary uses. It contains plant compounds that offer protection against inflammation and cancer, including cancers of the breast, and respiratory and digestive tracts. Some compounds in olive oil may even help control certain cancers once they have already developed.

Contrary to popular belief, it's fine to cook with olive oil, as it contains compounds like polyphenols, tocopherols, and monounsaturated fats that protect against damage caused by heat. Nonetheless, it's best not to heat it above 400°F, as this can reduce the oil's beneficial compounds. We suggest you use as little oil as possible during cooking and drizzle more over the finished dish, as is the custom in many Mediterranean countries.

Other fats that are well suited to cooking at higher temperatures include coconut oil, ghee (clarified butter), and refined avocado oil.

Minimize These Fats:

- Industrially refined seed oils, such as soybean, canola, corn, grapeseed, sunflower, safflower, and cottonseed oil, and any processed foods with these. These oils contain high concentrations of omega-6 fatty acids and undergo heavy processing, which removes their natural nutrients.

- Trans fats. These are manmade, partially hydrogenated vegetable oils found in commercial baked goods, fried foods (such as donuts and chips), frying fats, vegetable shortening, and margarine.

Over to You: Healthy Fats Action Plan

- Clean out your pantry. Take a close look at the food labels in your fridge and pantry. If they contain the words *soybean, canola, sunflower, safflower, cottonseed, corn*, or *hydrogenated*, discard them. And get rid of processed foods that contain these oils, such as mayonnaise, ready-made salad dressings, oil sprays, margarine, vegetable shortening, prepared meals, cake and cookie mixes, and anything that claims it tastes like butter (but isn't).
- Check the "best by" dates on any cooking and baking oils, nuts, seeds, and nut butters; if they've expired, discard them.
- Replace the oils you discard with healthy fats: extra virgin olive oil, coconut oil, and grass-fed, organic ghee. When buying avocado oil, be selective; a study by researchers at the University of California, Davis that appeared in the journal *Food Control* in October 2020 found that 82% of avocado oils sold in the U.S. are adulterated. We recommend avocado oil products made by Chosen Foods (chosenfoods.com), one of only two brands that passed the test.
- Omega-3-rich oils, such as flax, hemp, or walnut oil, should only be used cold and stored in a fridge or freezer.
- Buy unsweetened nut butters (almond, hazelnut) or seed butters (tahini, sunflower, pumpkin) in

small jars. Make sure they don't contain palm oil or other added ingredients.

- Buy unsalted, raw nuts (almonds, walnuts, pecans, hazelnuts, Brazils, macadamias) and seeds (pumpkin, flax, hemp, sunflower, sesame, pine kernels); store in a dark, cool place
- Make your own salad dressing using olive oil. Check out the Mediterranean vinaigrette recipe on Conner's website, modernmediterranean.com.
- For a few days, track your meals on a food journaling app like Cronometer to see how much fat you're eating. Aim to obtain around 35–40% of the calories you eat from healthy fats (if you're eating a keto diet, you'll aim for fat intakes closer to 75–80%).

If you need to increase your intake of healthy fat, drizzle a little olive oil over your food, make sauces, dips and dressings with nut and seed butters, sprinkle nuts, seeds, feta or goat cheese over your salad, snack on nuts and seeds, eat plenty of oily fish (e.g., salmon, mackerel, sardines) and carry small sachets of unsweetened nut butter with you as emergency snacks.

Know Your Carbs: The Insulin Connection

Carbohydrates are one of the most controversial topics in the context of cancer and nutrition. The body likes carbohydrates because they provide glucose, a ready source of energy for every cell in the body. But cancer cells also thrive on glucose, and to make matters worse, the hormones that get secreted when glucose levels rise—insulin and IGF-1—can further drive cancer growth.

So, should you eat carbohydrates or avoid them like the plague? We recommend the middle path: eating a moderate amount of nutrient-dense, low-glycemic carbohydrates while limiting refined, processed carbs.

Your body handles all carbohydrates the same way: Digestion converts them into glucose (blood sugar) for energy. Glucose in the bloodstream stimulates the pancreas to release the regulating hormone insulin.

If there is excess glucose—for instance, after eating a big plate of pasta—this gets stored in the liver and muscles as glycogen. When glycogen stores are full, insulin converts the remaining glucose and deposits it in the body's fat cells. This is how refined carbohydrates drive body fat gain: They spike blood glucose, triggering a release of insulin which, in turn, converts the glucose into body fat.

Eventually, your liver, muscles and fat cells are "full" and no longer want to take up glucose, no matter how loudly insulin urges them to. This state is called "insulin resistance," where the pancreas produces insulin but the body's cells do not respond (they resist the effects of insulin). Thus, the glucose cannot get into these cells and remains in the bloodstream. This prompts the pancreas to pump out more insulin to try to get the glucose into the body's cells. As a result, insulin levels rise; this leads to a state of chronically elevated insulin levels, called hyperinsulinemia.

Other, non-dietary factors also contribute to elevated insulin, such as a sedentary lifestyle; chronic stress; poor sleep; inflammation; environmental chemicals; certain medications; genes; imbalanced gut bacteria; a high intake of alcohol, nicotine or caffeine; and artificial sweeteners. Anyone with high insulin levels should consider these factors in addition to watching their dietary carbohydrate intake.

So, how does all this relate to cancer? Each time the pancreas secretes insulin, the liver releases a closely related chemical called insulin-like growth factor 1 (IGF-1). IGF-1 stimulates cells to grow—including cancer cells. Insulin and IGF-1 also fuel inflammation, which paves the way for tumor growth (for more on inflammation, see p. 174). Moreover, insulin and IGF-1 may strengthen the ability of abnormal cells to invade surrounding tissues. This is how high levels of circulating glucose, insulin, and IGF-1 fuel cancer growth.

Population studies bear this out:

- People with diabetes and prediabetes, who frequently have elevated blood glucose and insulin levels, are more prone to cancers of the colon, breast, prostate, liver, and pancreas than people with normal blood sugar levels
- Diets high in sugars and refined starches are also associated with ovarian, colorectal, breast, and pancreatic cancers
- Men with abnormally high IGF-1 levels have been found to have a four-fold higher risk of developing prostate cancer than men with normal levels, and insulin resistance is linked to earlier deaths in men with prostate cancer (see pubmed.ncbi.nlm.nih.gov/9438850)
- Women with insulin resistance have an increased risk of developing breast cancer—and a poorer prognosis once they have the disease—than women who are not insulin-resistant (see pubmed.ncbi.nlm.nih.gov/25404888)

Insulin resistance is associated with various cardiometabolic risk factors, such as low HDL ("good") cholesterol and high triglycerides, high blood pressure, fatty deposits in the liver, and high levels of systemic inflammation. When three or more of these risk factors are present, a person has a condition called "metabolic syndrome."

Worryingly, nearly 35% of all U.S. adults, and 50% of those 60 years of age or older, were estimated in 2011–2012 to have metabolic syndrome, and those numbers are rising. In people with obesity, the numbers are worse: insulin resistance can be found in over 50% of obese adolescents and 70% of obese women. Among adults with type 2 diabetes, the prevalence of insulin resistance rises to over 80%. Indeed, in 2018 researchers at the University of North Carolina at Chapel Hill estimated that a mere 12% of Americans are metabolically healthy (see pubmed.ncbi.nlm.nih.gov/30484738).

Do You Have Insulin Resistance?

Many people have no idea that they have insulin resistance. In most cases there are no obvious symptoms until they develop full-blown diabetes. However, there's an excellent way to test your insulin levels, and we believe anyone with a current or previous diagnosis of cancer should get it. Sadly, many doctors still don't know about it.

The "glucose tolerance test with insulin" (also called "insulin response to glucose test") is the most sensitive test to identify early-onset insulin resistance. The lab first draws some blood to measure your fasting glucose level and fasting insulin level. This test then measures both insulin and blood sugar after you ingest a 75-gram load of sugar (the equivalent of two sodas). If your doctor doesn't have or is unfamiliar with this test, you can order it directly from Dr. Lawenda's website: ioeprogram.com/lab-tests.

There's also a low-tech way to assess whether you might have insulin resistance, and this is by calculating your waist-to-height ratio (WHtR). To do this, measure your waist circumference (in inches/cm) with a tape measure (at the navel for men, an inch above the navel for women). Divide that number by your height (in inches/cm) and multiply it by 100. If the number is above the healthy range (42–48 for women, 43–52 for men), you may have insulin resistance. Ask your doctor to confirm this with a blood test.

If you have insulin resistance or diabetes, ask your doctor to prescribe a continuous glucose monitor, such as Dexcom (dexcom.com) or FreeStyle Libre (freestylelibre.us). This is the best way to track your real-time glucose levels in response to the foods and drinks you consume and other factors such as stress, sleep, exercise, and medications.

The Glucose Rollercoaster

Keeping glucose and insulin levels within a healthy range creates an environment in your body that's less conducive to cancer. One way you can influence the amount of insulin your pancreas secretes is to carefully select the amounts and types of carbohydrates you eat.

People who are metabolically healthy—generally, younger or physically active folks—can eat relatively generous amounts of carbohydrate without suffering adverse effects. However, people with cancer or metabolic syndrome usually do best when they limit carb intakes to around 15–25 grams of net carb per meal. Some people—for instance a person eating a ketogenic diet (see p. 165)—eat no more than 25–30 grams of carbohydrate per day.

Each of us is biochemically unique, which is why carbohydrate requirements vary from one person to another. Ask a nutrition professional to help you determine what level of carbohydrate intake is right for you.

Carb Quality Matters

The *amount* of carbohydrate you eat isn't the only determinant of your glucose, insulin, and IGF-1 levels. What type of carbohydrate you eat matters too.

In the 1980s, scientists devised a ranking system that rates carbohydrates according to their effect on blood glucose, called the glycemic index (GI). This system was further refined in the late 1990s, when nutrition researchers devised the concept of glycemic load (GL), which takes the quantity eaten into account. They came up with the following ranges:

- Low-glycemic (ideal): GI below 50; GL below 10
- Moderately glycemic (OK): GI of 50–70; GL of 10–20
- High-glycemic (minimize): GI above 70; GL above 20

When you eat a high-glycemic carbohydrate—for instance, a food that's sugary or starchy and low in fiber—this can push blood glucose sharply higher and trigger a hefty secretion of insulin, which in turn causes blood glucose to drop. This "sugar crash" can cause headaches, irritability, and cravings for more sugary or starchy foods. If you respond by eating a sugary snack, the surge-and-crash sequence starts over again. Over time, this blood-sugar roller coaster contributes to insulin resistance and all its associated problems.

This spike-and-crash sequence looks something like this:

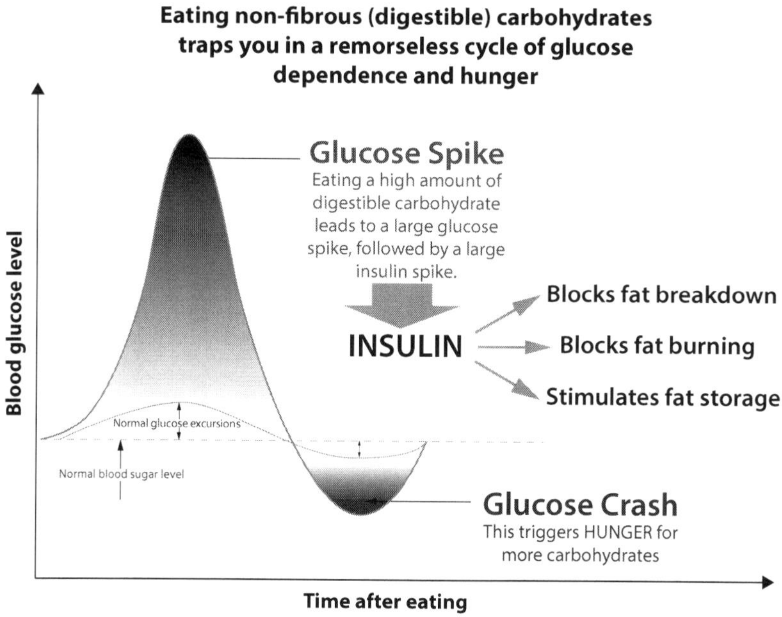

Figure 1: Dr. Ted Naiman, burnfatnotsugar.com

Eating carbohydrates that are minimally refined, contain fiber, and have a low or moderate glycemic rating (a.k.a. low-glycemic) on the other hand, can help maintain steady glucose, insulin, and IGF-1 levels.

Nutritious, low-glycemic carbohydrates are found in:

- Non-starchy vegetables like spinach, chard, kale, asparagus, leeks
- Legumes: chickpeas, lentils, whole and split dried peas, beans—ideally soaked and cooked from scratch
- Fruit, particularly those with lower sugar contents, such as berries, tart apples, oranges, grapefruit, peaches, plums, apricots
- Intact grains: oats (preferably as whole groats or steel-cut), barley, bulgur, quinoa

Less nutritious, high-glycemic carbohydrates include:

- Sugar and sugary foods (candy, sugar-sweetened soda, sweet confections)

- Baked goods made with white flour (breads, bagels, donuts, cookies, etc.)
- Most commercial, boxed breakfast cereals and instant oatmeal
- White rice (especially sushi rice)
- Pasta (especially gluten-free, like rice noodles or corn pasta)
- Fruit juice
- Some foods generally considered healthy, like raisins, sports drinks, rice cakes, corn flakes, baked potatoes

Oregon State University has posted a list of the glycemic loads of the most commonly eaten foods at extension.oregonstate.edu/sites/default/files/documents/1/glycemicindex.pdf. And if you're searching for something that's not listed here, look it up on glycemicindex.com, the biggest GI/GL database.

This system isn't 100% foolproof; studies show that people can have different glucose responses to the same foods. However, if you can't get a continuous glucose monitor that shows you exactly how you respond to specific foods, focusing on eating more low-glycemic foods and limiting high-glycemic foods is a good place to start.

Glycemic Damage Control

There may be times when you have no choice but to eat a higher-glycemic food—for instance, when traveling or eating a meal someone else has prepared for you. In this case, you can moderate the blood sugar reaction in various ways:

Limit the serving size. In any one meal, try to eat no more than:

- one slice of bread (if you can, choose sourdough, which is less glycemic than yeast-leavened bread),
- 1/2 pita bread,
- 1/2–3/4 cup cooked rice,
- 1/2–3/4 cup cooked pasta (equivalent to 1½–2 oz dry pasta),
- 2 small boiled potatoes,

- 1/2 medium baked potato (with skin), or
- 3–4 crackers

Accompany carbohydrates with fiber, protein, and fat to slow the speed at which your stomach empties and the carbs converts into blood glucose. For instance, when you eat rice, accompany it with chicken (protein) cooked in coconut milk (fat) with vegetables or chickpeas (fiber). Other examples: a moderate serving of pasta (carbs) with a generous helping of meat sauce (protein and fat) and a mixed salad with olive oil vinaigrette (fat and fiber), or a slice of sourdough toast (carb) with tuna salad (protein and fat) and a handful of sugar snap peas (fiber).

Add something acidic. The more acid a carb-rich meal contains, the lower its glycemic impact. For example, sourdough bread, which contains lactic acid, has a lower GL than white bread. The GL of freshly cooked potatoes can be as high as 24, but when coated with a vinegar-and-oil dressing and refrigerated for 24 hours, their GL drops to 13. Other ways to add acidity: Add tomatoes to pasta sauce. Flavor dishes with lemon juice, yogurt, or sour cream. Drink kombucha, kefir, or water with added lemon juice or apple cider vinegar alongside your meal. Have salads dressed in vinaigrette (oil and vinegar) with your meals.

Add foods, herbs, and spices that lower the glycemic impact of high-GI carbohydrates: these include oily fish, green tea, cocoa, foods rich in vitamin E such as nuts and avocado, spices like cinnamon, ginger, and fenugreek, and vegetables like okra, garlic, and onion.

Walk it off: When you use your muscles, even gently, you burn blood glucose. One study found that a mere 10-minute walk after meals could lead to a 22% decrease in glucose (see pubmed.ncbi.nlm.nih.gov/27747394).

Delay eating carbs until the end of the meal: One study found that white bread and fruit juice consumed *after* meat and vegetables were significantly less glycemic than when they were eaten at the start of a meal (see pubmed.ncbi.nlm.nih.gov/26106234).

Consider Glucose-Balancing Supplements

Many natural plant compounds are effective in regulating blood sugar levels. Do not take any of these without first discussing it with your healthcare providers.

- Cinnamon: 120–6,000 mg per day; the Ceylon variety is superior to cassia
- Curcumin: 500 mg, morning and evening
- Berberine: 500 mg, morning and evening
- Alpha-lipoic acid: 300–1,800 mg per day, in divided doses
- Chromium picolinate: 1,000 mcg per day, in divided doses
- American ginseng: 100–200 mg per day, or 3,000 mg taken before a high-glycemic meal
- Milk thistle: 200 mg three times per day
- Inulin: start with 1–2 g once a day with at least 8 oz of water, for 2–3 weeks. After that, increase dose by 1–2 g, waiting another 2–3 weeks to adjust. The maximum dose is 5–7 g daily.
- Fenugreek: 5–50 g per day
- White mulberry: 1 g three times per day
- Glucomannan: start with 1 or 2 g per day with at least 8 oz of water, 30–45 minutes before a meal. Do this for 2–3 weeks. After that, increase dose by 1–2 g, waiting another 2–3 weeks to adjust. The maximum dose is 4 g daily.

Which Sugar Is Best?

We are often asked which type of sugar is the healthiest: Honey? Agave? Brown, date, or coconut sugar?

Alas, no sugars—even the fashionable ones—nourish our bodies; they should therefore be limited. In fact, the American Heart Association suggests limiting the amount of added sugar to 6 tsp (24 grams or 100 calories) a day for women and 9 tsp (36 g or 150 calories) for men. (This relates only to added sugars, not sugars that occur naturally in fruits, vegetables or dairy.) To put that into perspective, a 12-oz can of Coke contains 140 calories from sugar, while a regular-sized Snickers bar contains 120 calories from sugar.

Sugars and sweeteners make many foods taste delicious, and since we want you to enjoy your food, we're not saying you should banish all sweetness from your diet; we simply want to help you manage sugar intake so that it doesn't undermine your health.

Here are some suggestions for ways to manage sugar and sweeteners in your diet:

- **Get to know the sugars in food.** To tell if a processed food contains added sugars, look at the list of ingredients. Sugar has many names. Besides those ending in "ose," such as maltose or sucrose, sugar often hides under healthy-sounding (or downright mysterious) names like agave nectar, barley malt, beet sugar, blackstrap molasses, brown rice sugar, buttered syrup, cane juice, caramel, coconut sugar, corn sweetener, date sugar, dextran, malt syrup, panela, honey, and fruit juice concentrates. (In fact, sugar has 56 different names; see here: robertlustig.com/56-names-of-sugar/.) Logging foods on Cronometer will reveal their sugar content.
- **Read labels.** When choosing processed foods like flavored yogurts, granola bars, or breakfast cereals, check the nutrition information label to see how much added sugar a serving contains. If it approaches or exceeds your recommended daily allowance (24 g for women and 36 g for men; see above), consider eating less than a full serving.
- **Analyze and tweak.** Track your meals on a food-journaling app like Cronometer for a few days to identify how much sugar you consume. If it's more than your daily recommended maximum, identify which foods contain these sugars. Then make a plan to slowly reduce your intake. For example, over several weeks reduce the teaspoons of sugar in your coffee from three to two, to one, to none. Or learn to like dark chocolate, starting with 50% cocoa content, then 60%, next 65%,

75%, and eventually 80% or even 90%. After a while, the sugary foods you used to love will taste cloyingly sweet.

- **Eat whole, fresh fruits.** Fruit contains fiber and other components that can mitigate sugar's impact. Moreover, fruit sugar (fructose), while unhealthy in large quantities, has a weak impact on blood sugar and thus doesn't increase insulin or IGF levels. Even so, consume fruits in moderation. Fruits nowadays are bred for sweetness and contain more sugar than they did 50–100 years ago.
- **Use honey or maple syrup in moderation.** The most natural source of sugar is honey, which has some antioxidant, anti-microbial, tumor-killing, and anti-inflammatory properties. Use raw honey that has not been heat-treated. Pure maple syrup has a lower glycemic impact than honey and undergoes little refining. Both are concentrated sugars, however, so limit your intake and accompany, where possible, with protein and fat (for instance, a teaspoon drizzled over yogurt).
- **Minimize agave.** Agave syrup is derived from plants but, unlike honey, it undergoes heavy processing. Worse still, it contains as much as 90% fructose, a type of sugar that contributes to fatty liver disease, weight gain, and insulin resistance.
- **Moderate keto sweeteners.** Xylitol and erythritol are so-called sugar alcohols extracted from plant sources (they don't contain actual alcohol). They are significantly lower in calories than sugar and have no effect on blood sugar, which is why they are popular among people eating low-carb and ketogenic diets. However, some of these sweeteners can cause bloating and GI discomfort, so, if you want to try them, start with small amounts and increase gradually. Other low-carb sweeteners, like monk fruit sweetener, stevia and allulose, are gentler on the digestive tract. Ultimately, however, we recommend that you limit even these low-carb sweeteners as little

as possible. For one, we lack long-term studies about their safety. Moreover, eating large amounts of keto-sugar-sweetened foods will keep your sweet tooth alive and kicking and fueling sugar cravings.

- **Enjoy nutritious desserts.** Eat berries, dark chocolate mousse, or two to three squares of dark chocolate (minimum 75% cocoa content) for dessert. Save fancy desserts—cakes, ice creams, etc.—for special occasions. Check Conner's website, modernmediterranean.com, for delicious low-carb and keto dessert recipes.
- **Brush and floss right away.** An effective strategy for preventing after-dinner snacking is to thoroughly brush and floss your teeth as soon as the meal is over. Studies have also found that eating adequate protein can lower late-night sugar and carb cravings.
- **Sleep to prevent cravings.** When you feel fresh and rested in the morning after 7–8 hours' sleep, you're less likely to need to climb aboard the blood sugar roller coaster (coffee, sweet pastries, sugary cereals, day-long snacking...).

Metformin and Berberine—More Than Blood-Sugar Treatments?

Blood sugar and insulin play a key role in a wide variety of cancers, so, it's not surprising that diabetes treatments could help with cancer prevention and treatment.

Metformin, derived from the herb *Galega officinalis*, has been used for over 50 years for diabetes management. Metformin is FDA approved only for diabetes, but this may change as evidence emerges about its anticancer effects. In fact, more than 100 clinical trials are in process, investigating its use in cancer treatment and prevention. Discuss with your primary care provider or endocrinologist whether to take metformin.

Metformin:

- Reduces blood sugar; cancer loves sugar, so reducing the sugar available to feed cancer cells may slow their growth
- Kills cancer stem cells, often the most treatment-resistant cell type in tumors
- May prevent precancerous cells from evolving into cancer cells
- Reduces the amount of circulating estrogen and testosterone, both of which can stimulate the growth of hormone-dependent tumors
- Provides anti-angiogenic properties, pro-apoptotic effects, and reduces activation of tumor growth signaling pathways
- Increases the anticancer effectiveness of certain chemotherapy drugs, such as paclitaxel, carboplatin, and doxorubicin
- May block other metabolic pathways that cancer cells depend on for survival and growth

Berberine, traditionally used in Ayurvedic, Chinese, and Native American medicines, is a non-prescription alternative to metformin because it exerts many of the same effects. Do not take berberine without first discussing it with your primary care provider.

Berberine:

- Protects the liver against chemotherapy injury
- Increases the effectiveness of radiation therapy and chemotherapy
- Offers anti-inflammatory, anti-angiogenic, and antidepressant effects
- Causes cancer cell death
- Slows cancer growth
- Inhibits the development of cancer from carcinogen exposure
- Shows anticancer activity against brain tumors (glioma) and cancers of the breast, head, and neck, leukemia,

liver cancer, lung cancer, melanoma, neuroblastoma, ovarian cancer, pancreatic cancer, prostate cancer, stomach cancer, and thyroid cancer
- Makes tumor cells more vulnerable to radiation therapy while protecting normal cells
- Protects cancer cells from becoming drug resistant by inhibiting the cellular membrane proteins that pump drugs out of the cells, and works synergistically with other chemo drugs to enhance cancer cell death

Over to You: Carbohydrate Action Plan

- **Track your carb intake.** Use the Cronometer food-journaling app for a short period of time to identify how much carbohydrate you consume. Aim for 50–100 g net carbohydrate per day; set your optimal target with the help of a nutrition professional.
- **Monitor glucose levels.** A simple blood sugar monitor is a great start, but a continuous glucose monitor will provide much more detailed information. Ask your doctor to prescribe one for you.
- **Eat out wisely.** At restaurants, avoid highly glycemic foods. For instance, at a sushi bar, order sashimi (fish without rice) rather than sushi (and don't eat raw fish at all if your white blood cell count is low). Decline the bread basket. At Indian, Thai, or Chinese restaurants, avoid noodle dishes, and if eating rice, have no more than a 1/2 cup rice (preferably brown) and fill up on fish, meat, and vegetables.
- **Eat fiber-rich foods.** Fiber helps to control the rise of blood sugar after a meal. If you eat a high-glycemic carbohydrate (such as pizza), accompany it with a fiber-rich side dish (like a large salad of mixed greens or beans).

Mighty Micronutrients

The three macronutrients—protein, fats, and carbohydrates—make up the bulk of the human diet. But micronutrients—vitamins, minerals, and other bioactive compounds found especially in plant foods—are every bit as important. Although you only need them in minuscule amounts, these "magic wands" facilitate the hundreds of reactions needed for proper body function.

Unfortunately, many people in the United States and other developed countries don't consume enough micronutrients. These inadequacies even occur when micronutrient intakes are above "deficiency" level (the Recommended Daily Allowance, or RDA) but below dietary intake recommendations. Micronutrient inadequacies increase the risk for many chronic diseases, including cancer.

Use micronutrient testing, such as the Genova NutrEval micronutrient assay, to determine your levels of vitamins, minerals, amino acids, and fatty acids. Retest again three to six months later. To obtain this test, contact your healthcare provider, consult a functional medicine provider, or order it through Dr. Lawenda's website: ioeprogram.com/lab-test.

If you need to add micronutrients to your current diet or supplementation regime, consult an expert, one who understands this may support or hinder your treatment and recovery. People trained to advise you on supplements include integrative physicians, nutrition professionals, some nurses and nurse practitioners, and naturopathic physicians.

Always discuss all supplements with your healthcare provider before and while taking them.

Antioxidants During Cancer Treatment

In 2008, Dr. Lawenda and his colleagues published a review article for the *Journal of the National Cancer Institute* on antioxidants during cancer treatment (see pubmed.ncbi.nlm.nih.gov/18505970). The conclusions remain unchanged more than 10 years later:

- Although most studies do not show that antioxidants protect tumors from the effects of chemotherapy or radiation, a small number of animal and cell studies show a reduced efficacy of radiation therapy and chemotherapy.
- No *human* studies have reported reduced efficacy of either chemotherapy or radiation therapy when administered at the same time as antioxidants. (Exception: smokers who took vitamin E and beta-carotene during head and neck cancer radiation therapy.)

Depending on various factors, Dr. Lawenda usually recommends one of two possible approaches:

- **Cautious Approach:** Avoid high-dose antioxidants during chemotherapy and radiation therapy. Consuming your antioxidants through food and beverages or low-dose supplements (not exceeding the RDA) is not likely to offer any significant protection to tumors. Antioxidant supplements for which there are no established RDAs (such as epigallocatechin-3-gallate (EGCG), the antioxidant in green tea, and curcumin) should either be consumed in moderation only in their whole-plant forms (green tea instead of EGCG extract, turmeric instead of curcumin), or avoided.
- **Less Cautious Approach:** Consider taking various antioxidant supplements (along with fruits and vegetables) to improve treatment tolerance and quality of life. Work with a provider who is highly knowledgeable in the safety of these supplements and their potential interactions with conventional treatments. Consider targeted intake, preferably through foods, of antioxidant micronutrient deficiencies. Before starting any new supplement, always discuss it with your oncology team.

While it may be safe to resume higher-dose antioxidants after the completion of chemotherapy or radiation therapy, these may lead to enhanced cancer-cell survival. Furthermore, some studies suggest that high-dose antioxidant supplements may increase the risk of certain cancers. Always talk with your oncology team before taking any supplement.

Vitamin C in Cancer Care

Test tube and animal studies support the role of vitamin C in cancer prevention, thanks to its antioxidant activity, its anti-inflammatory activity, and because it can block tumor initiation and promotion. The data for vitamin C and cancer risk in humans is mixed, however. Discuss with your doctor these vitamin C points:

- **Reduction of side effects.** Oral intake or IV administration of vitamin C may reduce side effects associated with cancer therapy. By decreasing side effects, vitamin C may increase the tolerance to cancer treatments, which should translate to improved outcomes.
- **Effect on cancer therapies.** No human studies have demonstrated an increased or decreased efficacy of cancer therapies when co-administered with oral or IV vitamin C (although many preclinical studies show synergistic effects). Be aware of this potential risk before choosing vitamin C therapy.
- **Ongoing research.** High-dose IV vitamin C, the most promising anticancer form of ascorbic acid, appears to be tolerable and safe based on small, pilot clinical studies. Numerous clinical trials are currently exploring the safety, tolerability, dosing, and potential efficacy of vitamin C in cancer patients.

Over to You: Micronutrient Action Plan

- Ask your doctor to test your micronutrient status, especially if you have been eating a diet high in processed or refined foods or have trouble digesting and absorbing your food

- If you have any nutrient deficiencies, consult with a nutrition professional to learn how to eat more of the foods that contain the nutrients you need
- Ask your doctor about any supplements you might need
- Talk to your doctor about antioxidant or vitamin C therapy

Prioritize Plant Foods

A diet rich in plant foods provides thousands of phytochemicals (plant chemicals) with a multitude of cancer-protective properties. Some, like cabbage and citrus, help the body eliminate toxic molecules that could kick-start the development of cancerous cells. Others, such as green tea, may act at a later stage by preventing the formation of new blood vessels tumors need to grow. A few—for instance, berries—are thought to intervene at nearly every stage of cancer development.

You don't have to memorize which food does what; all you need to remember is: *Eat whole plant foods*. Lots of different ones. Every day. At every meal.

Valorous Vegetables. Vegetables should appear on your plate every day, at every meal—at least five, and ideally 10 servings a day. The more colorful and flavorful, the better. For main meals, at least half of your plate should be taken up with vegetables. Potatoes and corn don't count as vegetables, but other starchy vegetables, such as parsnips and sweet potatoes, do (though since these are high in carbohydrate, enjoy them in moderation).

Fabulous Fruit. The best way to eat fruit is the way it comes off the tree or bush: raw, fresh, and whole. Dried fruit is an excellent source of fiber but loses many of its vitamins during dehydration and can push your blood glucose sharply higher, because it contains concentrated sugars, so limit this. Fruit juice isn't a nutritious choice; without whole fruits' natural fiber, fruit juice is essentially sugar water.

Every. Single. Day. If you think eating five to 10 servings of vegetables and fruits a day sounds impossible, here's how to get it done. (One serving is a piece of fruit or a pile of vegetables the size of your fist.)

Breakfast:

- A smoothie made with plain yogurt, almond butter, and 1 cup strawberries (two fruit servings)
- 3 oz spinach braised in olive oil with garlic (one vegetable serving), topped with two poached eggs, accompanied by a small apple (one fruit serving)
- Bircher muesli (overnight oats) containing 1/2 large apple (grated) and topped with 1/2 cup berries (two fruit servings)

Lunch:

- Greek salad with feta cheese, one tomato or seven cherry tomatoes, a pile of chopped lettuce, a 3-inch piece of cucumber, and two chopped spring onions (three vegetable servings)
- Large mixed salad of lettuce, tomatoes, onions, cucumber, celery, cubed apple, avocado, and beans, topped with fish, chicken, or hard-boiled egg (three vegetable servings)
- Bowl of mixed vegetable minestrone with chicken sausage (two to three vegetable servings)

Afternoon snack:

- An apple, orange, or tangerine with a handful of almonds (one fruit serving)
- 1/2 cup sugar snap peas with 1/4 cup roasted bell pepper dip (mouhammara) (two vegetable servings)

Dinner:

- Fish or chicken in tomato sauce with lentils and braised spinach (two and a half vegetable servings)
- Fish/meat with spaghetti squash, green beans, cauliflower, or spinach (non-starchy substitutes for pasta, rice, or potato) (one to two vegetable servings)

- Sheet-pan salmon with roasted onions, peppers, eggplants, and green beans (two vegetable servings)

At any point in the day:

- 8 oz tomato or other vegetable juice (one vegetable serving)

Eat the Rainbow. Different plant chemicals give fruits and vegetables their colors. Red and pink fruits and vegetables, such as tomatoes, watermelon, or pink grapefruit, provide lycopene, an antioxidant compound that protects against prostate and lung cancers. Purple vegetables and fruits, such as blackberries, blueberries, red apples and pears, red cabbage and eggplant, are rich in anthocyanins and proanthocyanidins, antioxidant compounds thought to prevent the development of blood vessels in tumors and protect against gastrointestinal cancers.

Thankfully, you don't need to learn the biochemistry of every plant food on your plate; all you need to remember is to eat as many different-colored plant foods as possible, and to vary them with the changing seasons.

Frozen or fresh? If harvested, frozen, and stored under optimal conditions, frozen produce offers a similar nutritional profile as fresh. Plus, frozen veggies are cleaned and ready for use, cutting down on prep time and cost (you only pay for the edible portion). Stick to foods that are frozen without the addition of other ingredients, such as seasonings or sauces.

Plant All-Stars

We never tire of repeating: There is no single, miraculous "anticancer" food. It's the combination of fresh, nutritious foods that offers optimum protection. Some foods, however, have been more thoroughly researched than others in the context of cancer and found to have cancer-fighting properties:

Cruciferous veggies. People who eat a lot of cruciferous vegetables (those in the cabbage family) are considerably less likely to develop cancer than people who eat them rarely.

That's because these vegetables—also known brassicas—contain two powerful compounds that reduce the development and progression of cancer: sulforaphane and indole-3-carbinol (I3C).

Sulforaphane has multiple cancer-protective properties: It helps shut off genes that promote the transformation of abnormal cells into cancer cells; it reduces the number of cancer stem cells, considered the most difficult cancer cell type to eradicate; it induces cancer cell death, blocks the formation of tumor blood vessels, and suppresses cancer cell spread; and it helps to promote the excretion of carcinogens from the body.

Indole-3-carbinol (I3C) and its metabolite bis (3'-indolyl) methane (DIM) slow the growth of cancer cells and tumors by impairing cell cycle pathways, inducing cancer cell death, and blocking the formation of blood vessels to tumors.

Chewing releases a plant enzyme that creates sulforaphane and I3C, so chew raw crucifers thoroughly. When cooking, steam cruciferous vegetables for 2–3 minutes (crisp-tender, not soft) to make them easier to digest and to reduce thyroid-disrupting compounds. To preserve their cancer-protective nutrients, don't boil them.

Alliums. All the members of the allium family—garlic, onions, leeks, shallots, spring onions, and chives—may help prevent the onset or progression of certain types of cancers, especially stomach, colorectal, laryngeal, and esophageal cancers. Garlic's health effects are most powerful when raw garlic is crushed or chopped and left to sit for 5–10 minutes before use.

Mushrooms. The best-known medicinal mushrooms are Asian varieties such as oyster, maitake, shiitake, and reishi (lingzhi) mushrooms. Even everyday button mushrooms may have a protective effect: Researchers at Perth University found that Chinese women eating on average 4 g of dried button mushrooms daily cut their breast cancer risk by 47% compared to women eating none, while those eating 10 g of fresh mushrooms daily lowered their risk by 64%. Those who combined mushrooms with regular green tea intake saw their breast-cancer risk decline by 89% (see pubmed.ncbi.nlm.nih.gov/19048616). Raw button mushrooms contain potentially carcinogenic compounds, though, so cook them before consumption.

Berries. Many of the compounds in berries offer protection against certain cancers. Ellagic acid, for example, found in raspberries and strawberries, may slow the growth and spread of tumors and aid the body in detoxifying potentially cancer-causing substances. The best way to eat berries is fresh and raw, but frozen berries are also fine.

Citrus. Studies suggest that eating citrus fruits—including lemons, oranges, grapefruit, limes, and tangerines—lowers the risk of certain cancers, especially those along the digestive tract. Protective factors in citrus juice and peel may help remove potentially carcinogenic substances from the body and inhibit cancer cell growth. Stock a basic supply of organic citrus fruit and add juice and/or zest to salad dressings, sauces, stews, fish dishes, and desserts. (The peel of conventionally grown citrus may contain toxic chemicals; only use the zest of untreated citrus fruits.)

Over to You: Plant Food Action Plan

- If you never eat vegetables or fruits, start with one a day and increase gradually
- Aim to eat at least five—and preferably closer to 10—servings of vegetables and fruits per day
- Eat more vegetables than fruits (some items that, botanically, are fruits qualify as vegetables here, such as tomatoes, eggplant, green beans, squash, okra, olives, avocados, and cucumbers)
- If you have trouble eating or digesting vegetables, blend them (blending vegetables and fruits in a high-powered blender, rather than juicing them, retains their precious fiber)

- You may enjoy certain vegetables served in restaurants; if so, look up the recipe online and try making it at home
- Look for tasty vegetable recipes in Conner's book, *Zest for Life: The Mediterranean Anticancer Diet*, or her website, modernmediterranean.com

Juicing and Blending

Whole vegetables and fruits are your best source of nutrition, but juicing and blending these can be a boon for people undergoing cancer treatment, because they provide hydration and nutrients quickly and easily. Think of juices and smoothies as the ultimate anti-cancer supplement.

Juicing (which pulverizes and squeezes produce, extracting juice and discarding fiber) and blending (which finely chops the plant material and retains the fiber, producing smoothies) enable you to consume your recommended intake of vegetables and fruits without spending hours preparing, chewing, and digesting them—a formidable task when your appetite and digestive capacities are battered by cancer treatment. A single 12-ounce glass of juice can pack in 2–3 lbs' worth of concentrated nutrients, more than most people could eat in a day. Best of all, you achieve powerful nutrient synergies, because you obtain the plants' healthful compounds in the same proportions as if you had eaten them.

One of the benefits of blending is that you eat the whole plant food, including its fiber, which is likely to cause a less pronounced increase in blood glucose than drinking juice. On the other hand, for an individual who has been advised by their doctor to eat a low-fiber diet, fresh juice may be easier to digest than a fiber-rich vegetable smoothie.

Equipment

If you plan to use your blender more than a couple of times per week, get one that's powerful, durable, easy to clean, and

BPA-free. Our favorite brands are Blendtec and Vitamix. They're more expensive than other blenders, but it's a worthwhile investment, as they produce much smoother juices and are fantastic for making milks and butters from nuts and seeds.

If you plan to make juice, opt for a masticating juicer, which uses an auger (gears) to slowly grind and crush vegetables and literally squishes out the juice. This will give you a higher nutrient content than a centrifugal juicer. If you're looking for a juicer that processes vegetables and fruit equally well, works quickly, and is easy to clean, get a vertical single-auger juicer. (Important caveat: these don't juice leafy greens such as wheatgrass very efficiently.) If you mainly want to juice vegetables and leafy greens, get a horizontal single-auger or double-auger juicer.

Juicing and Blending Tips:

- **Vary vegetables and fruits.** Varying your fruits and vegetables provides you with the broadest possible range of nutrients. It also reduces exposure to compounds that can cause problems when eaten in excess. For example, repeatedly adding only spinach or chard to your juices or smoothies could increase your risk of developing kidney stones, as these greens are high in oxalic acid; instead, rotate them with low-oxalic greens like kale, mustard greens, collards, dandelion, and arugula.
- **Drink juices and smoothies on an empty stomach.** This allows the vitamins and minerals to go straight to your bloodstream. Wait at least two hours after a meal to drink your juice. Wait 20 minutes after drinking a juice or smoothie to eat a meal.
- **Don't make juices or smoothies too far in advance.** When exposed to air, plant enzymes and nutrients begin to degrade. Drink your juice/smoothie within 15 minutes of making it.
- **If you need to drink it later, store in an airtight container.** Add some vitamin C (lemon or orange

juice or some powdered ascorbic acid or vitamin C supplement) to protect against oxidation. Fill the container to the top, leaving no air gap. Refrigerate no longer than 24 hours.

- **Don't use too many sweet fruits and vegetables.** Juicing produce with high sugar content can cause a rapid rise in blood sugar and an insulin spike. Use no more than one sweet fruit or vegetable (watermelon, apples, pears, carrots, and beets) per serving.
- **Keep things cold during juicing or blending.** Heat generated when making juice or smoothies may break down the natural enzymes in vegetables and fruits. To reduce heat, use cold produce; do not overload your juicer (feed in a little produce at a time); chop your produce into smaller pieces so the juicer doesn't have to work so hard; occasionally include an ice cube (this will thin the juice a little); replace dull blades or cutters; and juice in small batches.

Over to You: Juicing & Blending Action Plan

- If you don't own a juicer or a blender, decide which you'd get more use from and invest in the best-quality machine you can afford; look out for appliance sales or second-hand bargains
- Experiment with different combinations of fruits and vegetables, fresh or frozen
- Limit sweet fruits or vegetables to one per serving
- Add fresh ginger or turmeric root for an extra boost of anticancer compounds
- Add a teaspoon of extra virgin olive oil to your juice to enhance the absorption of fat-soluble vitamins; if you're trying to gain weight, add even more

Spice Up Your Health

For thousands of years our ancestors have appreciated herbs and spices, not only because they make food taste delicious but for their healing properties. Science now shows they have a wide range of antimicrobial, antifungal, antioxidant, anti-inflammatory, and cancer cell growth-inhibiting and detoxifying actions.

Here's how to integrate them easily into your daily diet:

- Sprinkle chopped parsley, cilantro, chives, basil, or dill over every meal you eat: soups, stews, salads, omelets, etc., and add to smoothies (check out Conner's recipes for guidance)
- To enjoy the freshest herbs, grow your own; even a windowsill or balcony can accommodate a small selection of herbs in pots or boxes; thyme, oregano, rosemary, basil and mint are particularly easy to grow
- To store fresh herbs, rinse them, shake them dry or spin them briefly in a salad spinner, wrap them loosely in a paper towel, place in a zip-top bag, and refrigerate; this will keep them fresh for up to a week
- When buying or harvesting more herbs than you need, wash, dry, chop, and freeze them in small containers; be sure to label them—frozen herbs all look alike!
- Turn extra herbs into a sauce or emulsion together with garlic, olive oil, lemon juice, and other spices (for instance, basil pesto, or Moroccan chermoula made with cilantro and mint—see recipes in Conner's book, *Zest for Life*); pack in a small jar and cover with a thin layer of olive oil; refrigerate or freeze
- Buy dried herbs and spices in small quantities and use up as quickly as possible; store in dry, dark, cool surroundings with lids tightly sealed

Try Curcumin

When Mother Nature designed curcumin, a powerful plant compound in the root turmeric, she gave it the ability to target an astonishing multitude of mechanisms that cancers need to develop, grow, and spread. Curcumin has been shown to:

- Inhibit cancer cell division and spread
- Promote cancer cell death
- Decrease cell growth
- Inhibit growth of blood vessels to tumors
- Reduce progression of precancerous lesions of the mouth, cervix, skin, and stomach
- Exert anticancer activity against numerous cancer types
- Block the inflammation-producing NF-kB protein (involved in almost every stage of cancer development, progression, and recurrence)
- Boost the effects of chemotherapy and radiation therapy
- Be completely nontoxic to normal cells
- Protect healthy tissues from radiation and chemotherapy injury

New research even suggests that curcumin (and other botanical compounds, including EGCG in green tea, resveratrol in grapes, and genistein in soy) can influence human genes in a way that bolsters anticancer defenses.

Did you catch that? The exciting new science of epigenetics indicates that certain lifestyle choices, including what you eat, can *turn on or turn off certain genes*, including cancer-promoting or cancer-blocking genes. Epigenetic modifications only require very small concentrations of a compound to have a significant impact on gene expression—which may explain how curcumin affects so many biological processes, despite being poorly absorbed into the blood.

The FDA considers curcumin to be a safe supplement, food additive, and spice, but talk to your doctor about potential side effects, drug interactions, and contraindications. For example, curcumin may exacerbate existing gallbladder disease or kidney stones, cause uterine stimulation (use caution during pregnancy), and increase bleeding risk for those taking blood thinners.

How to Use Curcumin

As with any supplement, discuss curcumin with your oncology team before you start taking it.

For cancer prevention, 400–500 mg curcumin per day is widely recommended. During and after cancer treatment, 800–3,000 mg per day appears to be safe (divided dose, with meals). Curcumin is rapidly cleared from the blood, so take it in divided doses throughout the day.

If you want to eat turmeric instead of taking curcumin, you need to consume approximately two tablespoons of turmeric powder to obtain 500 mg curcumin.

Keep in mind that oral curcumin is poorly absorbed. To maximize absorption, activate curcumin with:

- Heat: simmer turmeric in a meal, drink, or paste before eating
- Black pepper extract: taking curcumin with piperine, a black pepper extract, has been shown to increase curcumin absorption by 2000%
- Fatty foods: olive oil, avocado, fish oil, milk, seeds
- Quercetin-rich foods: onions, apples, broccoli, green leafy vegetables, peppers, green tea

Over to You: Curcumin, Herb & Spice Action Plan

- Make a delicious chai concentrate comprising fresh turmeric, ginger, and other spices that you can enjoy hot or chilled (see recipe on Conner's website, modernmediterranean.com)
- Cook a curry; some of our favorite Indian cookbooks include *Entice with Spice* and the *Indian Instant Pot Cookbook*

- Ask your doctor if a curcumin supplement is safe for you; if so, choose one that's well absorbed; it's worth paying extra for optimal absorption
- Buy a starter kit of Mediterranean herbs and spices: dried bay leaves, ground coriander, ground cumin, dill, garlic powder, ground ginger, ground cinnamon, herbes de Provence or Italian herb mix, oregano, paprika powder (plain and smoked), red pepper flakes, rosemary, sage, thyme, turmeric
- If you have a garden or balcony, grow fresh herbs

Love Legumes

Legumes (known in the UK as "pulses") are plants that produce seed pods, such as beans, lentils, chickpeas, and peas, and are a key ingredient of the Mediterranean diet.

Many legumes contain natural compounds that resemble a weak form of estrogen, which may protect against certain types of cancer—notably breast and prostate cancer. Because beans are high in fiber and protein, they promote feelings of fullness by slowing down digestion. Legumes are an excellent source of "resistant" starch that feeds our gut bacteria and helps protect colon cells. Moreover, despite their high starch content, beans are generally low-glycemic foods. They're also inexpensive and versatile.

In recent years legumes have gotten a bad rap from nutrition enthusiasts warning of the adverse effects of compounds called lectins, carbohydrate-binding proteins found in all plants, but particularly in raw legumes and whole grains.

Active lectins (in raw or undercooked foods) can indeed cause negative side effects. For instance, eating raw or undercooked kidney beans, which contain phytohemagglutinin, a type of lectin that can cause red blood cells to clump together, can produce nausea, vomiting, stomach upset, and diarrhea. Milder side effects include bloating and gas.

However, when beans are carefully prepared, there is no evidence of lectins contributing to health problems in most people. In fact, they perform a variety of beneficial functions in the body, including participating in our immune response; certain lectins are even being studied for their potential role in protecting us from cancer.

Traditional preparations of beans and grains—practiced for millennia in the Mediterranean region—include soaking, fermenting, sprouting, and cooking; these can inactivate most lectins.

When cooking beans from scratch, soak them thoroughly and cook them (ideally in a pressure cooker) until done. Canned beans are pressure-cooked and packaged in liquid, so they generally are also low in lectins. (Make sure you drain the beans of the canning liquid and rinse them thoroughly.) However, simmering raw beans at low heat (for instance, in a slow-cooker), or undercooking beans will not remove all of the lectins.

Another thing that puts many people off eating legumes is the intestinal gas they can cause. This happens when the bacteria in the gut digest the fibers and sugars in legumes. To reduce this effect:

- Before cooking, soak beans for 24–36 hours, with two or three changes of soaking water; rinse thoroughly and cook until soft (pressure-cooking legumes is faster and the best way to remove lectins)
- Add a strip of kombu (seaweed) to the bean cooking water
- Add vinegar after cooking to render legumes more digestible
- Cook beans with aniseed, fennel, or coriander seeds, savory, cumin, caraway, and turmeric
- Before you start eating, take a supplement that contains the enzyme alpha-galactosidase (found in Beano and many digestive enzyme preparations); it

breaks down raffinose, a sugar in beans that's linked to gas production

- During or after eating beans, sip a tea or infusion of fennel, aniseed, peppermint, coriander, or chamomile
- Take small mouthfuls; chew each mouthful 30–40 times to help predigest the beans
- Train your gut to better tolerate beans by eating them regularly; start with small amounts, and gradually increase consumption
- Anecdotal evidence suggests that lentils and garbanzos may be less "gassy" than other legumes

If you suffer from irritable bowel syndrome or SIBO (see p. 182), you may need to reduce your intake of high-fiber foods like beans until the underlying problem has been resolved.

Is Soy Safe?

For years experts have debated the safety of soy foods for people with cancer. Some argue that soy's estrogen-like compounds—particularly isoflavones—protect against certain cancers, notably hormone-dependent cancers of the breast and prostate. Others, however, argue that these estrogen-like compounds are harmful for breast cancer patients and survivors.

While early rodent studies indicated potential risks of soy consumption for people with estrogen sensitive cancers, researchers have more recently concluded that rodents are poor models for testing how isoflavones affect human biology, because they metabolize soy very differently from humans.

Research studies differ widely on soy's likely impact on cancer risk. These disparate findings may reflect the different types of soy foods studied, the time of life at which they are consumed (childhood or adulthood), the type of cancer under investigation, and individual differences in genetics, gut microbes, or overall diet. Most of the population studies concerning the consumption of soy foods have been performed in Asian populations; this raises some questions as to how applicable the results might be to non-Asian populations, since Asians are typically better able to convert soy isoflavones into potentially protective compounds in the gut than non-Asians.

Overall, however, population studies—even in non-Asians—consistently indicate there is no increased risk for breast cancer survivors who consume soy foods. Emerging research even suggests that soy foods may decrease the likelihood of breast cancer recurrence in women with a history of the disease.

We therefore believe it's safe to eat a little soy in the context of a plant-based, nutrient-rich diet, though we recommend that you consume no more than one serving a day and choose organic soy foods. Avoid processed soy protein isolates (found in protein powders, energy bars, and cereals) and burgers, patties, sausages, or other soy-based meat substitutes that are designed to mimic the taste of meat. Also, avoid soy isoflavone supplements, because they often contain excessive amounts of phytoestrogen. Ultimately, soy isn't a part of the traditional Mediterranean diet; if you don't like or tolerate it, there's no pressing need to eat it.

Fantastic Flax

If you're not a fan of soy, you can derive a lot of similar benefits (plus a few extra) from flaxseed.

Flax contains compounds called lignans that have a chemical structure similar to estrogen. Earlier, this led to fears that lignans could promote cancers fueled by excess estrogen, or could interfere with anti-estrogen cancer treatments. However, in animal studies, flaxseed, and lignans isolated from flaxseed, have been shown to reduce both estrogen-positive (ER+) and estrogen-negative (ER-) breast cancer and have not interfered with actions of breast cancer drugs. The few animal studies addressing other cancers have shown some reduction in inflammation, a decrease in the number and size of colon cancer tumors, and in the growth and spread of prostate cancer.

Flaxseed has several other benefits, too. As the American Institute of Cancer Research (AICR) points out on its website, flax is an excellent source of soluble fiber, which forms a gel in the digestive tract, slowing digestion and, thus, the rise in blood sugar and insulin after eating. (More on glucose and insulin on pp. 104–117)

Viscous fiber's actions in the gut may also help reduce circulating estrogen levels. Such effects could help explain why some studies link greater intake of soluble dietary fiber to lower breast cancer risk, according to the AICR.

Flaxseed also contains alpha-linolenic acid (ALA), a form of omega-3 fat that our bodies convert into an anti-inflammatory omega-3 fat called EPA (eicosapentaenoic acid). Only a small proportion of ALA is converted into EPA; yet, in animal and human studies, even moderate amounts of flaxseed have been shown to increase EPA levels, according to the AICR.

Further, flaxseed boasts phenolic acids that increase cells' antioxidant and anti-inflammatory defenses and may improve glucose metabolism, decrease insulin resistance, and alter the gut microbes, creating an environment in the body less likely to support cancer. Incidentally, the viscous fiber in flax—which forms a thick gel upon contact with water—can improve bowel motility by bulking and softening fecal matter and lubricating the intestines.

Lastly, flax contains gamma-tocopherol, one of eight compounds that make up vitamin E. According to the AICR, cell and animal studies suggest that gamma-tocopherol may provide even stronger anti-inflammatory protection than the more widely known alpha-tocopherol. In both cell and animal studies, gamma-tocopherol decreases cancer cell growth.

You can sprinkle flaxseed over yogurt and oatmeal, and stir it into smoothies. It can also be used in baking; studies have found it to be heat-stable when used to bake breads and muffins.

We recommend you buy whole, organic flaxseed and store it in the refrigerator; grind the required amount in a coffee grinder or food processor and use immediately. Flaxseed may decrease the absorption of medications, so take it one hour before or two hours after any prescription or nonprescription medicine.

Whole Grains

Intact (unprocessed) whole grains can provide a wide range of nutrients, including vitamin E, most B vitamins, magnesium, zinc, and cancer-protective plant chemicals such as saponins and lignans.

On a calorie-for-calorie basis, however, non-starchy vegetables and fruits provide more fiber than grains do, more vitamins and minerals, more satiety (you'll eat less and feel fuller), and better digestibility. Legumes, meanwhile, contain twice as much protein as do whole grains. So, if you eat grains, consume them in moderation and in their least-processed states.

Some people—notably those with celiac disease—do not tolerate grains that contain gluten, a protein in grains such as wheat, barley, farro, rye, spelt, and kamut. If you have digestive problems, ask your doctor to test you for celiac disease.

Fermenting, sprouting, soaking, and cooking can improve grains' digestibility. For instance, soak oat or barley flakes overnight in water or milk and cook them into a thick and comforting porridge in the morning. (For a low-carb alternative to oatmeal, make a creamy porridge of coconut flour, flax, and chia seeds.)

If you eat bread, choose sourdough bread that's been leavened for several days; sourdough is less glycemic and easier to digest than bread leavened with baker's yeast. (Or try grain-free breads; see Conner's website, modernmediterranean.com, for recipes.)

Over to You: Beans and Grains Action Plan

- If you never eat legumes, gradually introduce them into your diet, starting with one meal a week and slowly increasing
- To reduce lectins and improve digestibility, prepare legumes carefully, soaking and cooking them thoroughly
- Add small amounts of legumes to some of your favorite meat dishes; for instance, use lentils in Bolognese sauce, or red beans in chile con carne
- Easy, Mediterranean-friendly legume dishes include Italian minestrone, Spanish chickpea stew, split pea soup, or Indian *dal* (curried lentil stew)
- Keep a tub of chickpea hummus in your fridge and eat it as a dip with raw vegetables
- Scatter canned chickpeas or cannellini beans over salads or into soups
- Cook a porridge of whole oats that have been soaked overnight; whole or steel-cut oats cooked in chicken bone broth with mushrooms taste like risotto!
- Visit modernmediterranean.com to find recipes involving traditionally prepared legumes and grains, as well as grain-free bread, porridge, or pizza

Eat Meat Wisely

Another long-running debate in the context of cancer and diet is whether eating meat—especially red meat—increases our risk of cancer.

Although many studies report risks (especially from processed meat), others do not. That's in large part because observational studies—the type on which many health authorities base their recommendations—are not very reliable.

Having said this, a massive meta-analysis of 118 studies with more than six million participants, published in the *Annals of Internal Medicine*, caused a stir in late 2019 by concluding that, despite some evidence that red meat consumption might be harmful, the evidence wasn't strong enough to justify telling people to change their dietary habits. "The possible absolute effects of red and processed meat consumption on cancer mortality and incidence are very small, and the certainty of evidence is low to very low," the study's authors concluded (see pubmed.ncbi.nlm.nih.gov/31569214).

We are reluctant to condemn meat. For one, high-quality meat, such as organic, pastured beef, lamb, or pasture-raised chicken, can be an excellent source of nutrients that may protect against cancer, such as omega-3 fatty acids and conjugated linoleic acid. Moreover, meat provides high-quality, complete protein that supplies the body with all the amino acids it needs to function properly.

It doesn't take large servings of meat to cover a person's protein needs, whereas it can be hard to get all the amino acids they need from plant foods—especially if they're undergoing cancer treatment and their appetite is low. So, eating some meat—not too much, not too little—is probably cancer-neutral and might even be beneficial.

Cook With Care

How you cook and eat meat may matter more to your cancer risk than whether you eat it. Smoking meats and barbecuing, frying, or grilling meat at high temperatures creates potentially carcinogenic substances, including polycyclic aromatic hydrocarbons (PAHs) and heterocyclic amines (HCAs). Salting and curing meat and fish is also associated with increased cancer risk, notably stomach cancer.

Oven roasting, braising, and baking involve lower temperatures, so fewer HCAs are likely to form (though gravy made from meat drippings contains substantial amounts). Slow-cooking, stewing, boiling, or poaching takes place at about 212°F (100°C), creating negligible HCAs.

Marinating meat with spices and herbs reduces the formation of HCAs even at high temperatures. One study showed that beef steaks bathed for an hour in a marinade containing thyme, rosemary, red and black pepper, allspice, and chives and cooked at 400°F (204°C) had 88% lower HCA content than non-marinated meat.

If you want to be healthy without giving up meat, follow these five basic rules:

Choose meat from traditionally reared animals. Meat from animals that range freely on pastureland is rich in nutrients. In a 2009 comparison of grass-fed vs. grain-fed beef (see pubmed.ncbi.nlm.nih.gov/19502506), grass-fed beef was:

- Lower in total fat
- Higher in antioxidants beta-carotene and vitamin E
- Higher in the B vitamins thiamin and riboflavin
- Higher in calcium, magnesium, and potassium
- Higher in total omega-3 fatty acids
- Healthier in its omega-6 to omega-3 ratio (1.65 in grass-fed beef vs. 4.84 in grain-fed)
- Higher in conjugated linoleic acid (CLA), a potential cancer fighter
- Higher in vaccenic acid (which can be transformed into CLA)

Minimize processed meat. Healthy meat from pastured animals can be rendered unhealthy through processing, including traditional salting or smoking methods. Even organic bologna luncheon meat is preserved with nitrites, and smoked pastured ham contains PAHs. Processed meats may also contain the additive carrageenan, found to promote tumors in rodents.

Eat modest servings of meat. Americans eat an average of 8 oz (225 g) of meat each day—that's nearly 200 lbs (90 kg) a year, three times more than the American Institute for Cancer Research recommends. Their advice is to eat no more than three servings (12–18 oz) of cooked red meat per week. Buying high-quality pastured meat may automatically curb your consumption because it costs more; happily, you can eat less of it and still get the nutrients you need.

Always serve a salad or vegetables alongside meat. Vegetables contain protective compounds that can counteract any potentially harmful effects of cooked meat. They also provide bulk, so you'll fill up faster. Moreover, leafy greens such as kale, broccoli, and spinach are rich in calcium, which binds to the iron in meat that could otherwise increase colorectal cancer risk.

Make your own "cold cuts," such as sliced, home-cooked chicken breast, meatloaf (fortified with vegetables, herbs, and spices), or homemade beef jerky marinated in olive oil, herbs, and spices.

Over to You: Healthy Meat Action Plan

- When you plan your meals, prioritize plant foods; if you eat an omnivorous diet, include animal foods like meat, fish, seafood, eggs, or dairy to help cover your protein needs
- Calculate how much protein you need per meal (most people need around 20–30 g) and figure out how much meat that translates into; for instance, 3 oz of cooked chicken contains 28 g of protein; to find out the protein content of commonly eaten foods, go to modernmediterranean.com/protein-content-table
- Eat the best-quality meat, eggs, and dairy you can afford; grass-fed or organic animal foods are more nutritious and better for the environment than their factory-farmed equivalents; visit eatwild.com to find out where you can buy pastured meat, eggs,

and dairy products produced on farms that practice regenerative agriculture

- Cook meat as gently as possible to prevent the formation of carcinogens; if you barbecue or fry it at high temperatures, marinate it first
- Eat modest servings of meat with generous servings of vegetables, and use herbs, spices and healthy fats in their preparation

Dairy Do's and Don'ts

An estimated three-quarters of the world's adult population doesn't tolerate lactose (the sugar in milk), and doesn't consume dairy. It is therefore an optional food for humans.

Indeed, after reviewing over 100 studies on dairy, two eminent Harvard professors, Walter Willett and David Ludwig, recently wrote in *The New England Journal of Medicine* that there is little evidence to support the long-standing public health recommendation to consume three servings of dairy foods daily.

That's not to say you shouldn't ever have dairy foods; they provide health benefits for those with poor diet quality, especially children. However, for people who eat nutritious diets, dairy foods are unnecessary, the Harvard researchers write.

Dairy proponents say that minerals and vitamins in milk—notably calcium and vitamin D—as well as healthy bacteria in fermented dairy foods, may have a cancer-protective effect. Detractors, on the other hand, argue that hormones, saturated fats, and drug and pesticide residues in dairy, and its potential hormonal effects in the human body, increase cancer risks.

As with meat, the research relating to dairy and cancer is mixed. Milk consumption is linked to prostate cancer in men and endometrial cancer in women. Moreover, a high intake of calcium from dairy products may increase the risk of prostate cancer. In contrast, milk consumption may protect against colorectal cancer.

When it comes to breast cancer, the picture isn't clear. In a large study analyzing data collected over 11 years from approximately 320,000 European women, researchers found no consistent relationship between breast cancer and milk consumption (or meat and egg consumption, for that matter). Another large study found that dairy consumption—especially reduced-fat dairy products—actually lowered breast cancer risk.

However, as with other observation studies involving cancer and nutrition, it can be difficult to prove cause and effect. Furthermore, most studies focus on adults in middle age or later, whereas risk factors for cancer may extend back to childhood.

Dairy has been eaten around the Mediterranean for thousands of years. However, the dairy products we consume nowadays have very little in common with traditional Mediterranean cheese, kefir, and yogurt. Intensive farming practices have led to less healthy omega-6-to-3 ratios in dairy, lower concentrations of protective conjugated linoleic acid, and reduced antioxidant levels compared with pastured cows.

Moreover, since commercial dairy cows are pregnant for most of the time they are milked, dairy can contain a variety of growth-promoting factors such as estrogen and progestins that may increase cancer risk. Moreover, processing methods—such as ultra-high-temperature pasteurization or ultrafiltration to increase the protein content of milk—produce very different milk products than those humans have traditionally consumed.

If You Eat Dairy...

Based on all the points listed above, we recommend that you eat dairy sparingly. When you do consume it, try to eat dairy from animals that were organically reared or grass fed. If you have a hormone-sensitive cancer, choose reduced-fat or fat-free dairy products, as most bovine estrogens are found in the fatty portion of the milk.

In the Mediterranean region, goat and sheep's milk are frequently consumed (for instance, as feta cheese, halloumi, fresh cheese and yogurt). Their milks contain more calcium and protein than cow's milk, so a little goes a long way. Moreover, the estrogen content of goat's milk has been found to be significantly lower than that in cow's milk—including organic cow's milk. (No comparable data exists for sheep's milk.) Lastly, many people who don't tolerate cow's milk are better able to digest milk from goats and sheep.

Some dairy foods—for instance, plain yogurt and kefir—may even have cancer-protective properties. Studies link kefir, a fermented milk product that tastes like buttermilk, to a reduced risk of breast cancer and bladder cancer. Moreover, the short-chain fatty acids in fermented dairy foods have been found to induce apoptosis (cell death) in colorectal carcinoma cells and gastric cancer cells.

Lastly, if you eat dairy, avoid processed, sweetened products such as low-fat flavored yogurts, smoothies, and frozen yogurt. These are often loaded with sugar and contain thickeners, sweeteners, artificial flavorings, and other additives no body needs.

Plant "Milk"

Plant-based beverages, such as almond, hemp, macadamia, and oat "milks," are acceptable—with caveats. Plant-based beverages generally provide little protein and few nutrients, and some—notably those made from grains—contain sugar and carbohydrates that can push blood-sugar levels higher, as well as various additives to make these drinks taste and feel more like cow's milk.

Moreover, plant "milks" are almost always packaged in containers lined with a thin layer of plastic that may leach estrogen-like chemicals into the milk. Some also contain carrageenan, a seaweed extract linked with gastrointestinal inflammation and ulcerations in susceptible people.

When you buy plant milk, choose unsweetened beverages with the shortest possible list of ingredients. Better still, make your own—it's easy. (See recipe on Conner's website.)

It's OK to Go Without

If, after weighing the pros and cons, you choose not to consume any dairy foods, this poses no health risk. Humans are the only mammals that consume dairy long after weaning. Indeed, our ability to digest lactose (the sugar in milk) begins to decline after age two, the age at which, in nature, we would typically be transitioning from mother's milk to solid foods. Might this be Nature's way of telling us to lay off milk after infancy?

If you think you need dairy for bone strength, rest assured: in many parts of the world people drink no milk and nonetheless have healthy bones. Cruciferous vegetables, legumes, nuts, seeds and bone-in fish (e.g., canned salmon, sardines, mackerel and anchovies) are excellent sources of calcium and other bone-building nutrients.

Over to You: Your Dairy Action Plan

- Review your diet and assess how much dairy you consume; limit intake to one to two servings a day
- Eat minimally processed (unflavored and unsweetened) dairy foods; you can add fruits and a touch of maple syrup to plain yogurt, and herbs to plain cottage cheese
- Replace dairy products from conventionally reared animals with grass-fed/organic equivalents
- Try goat or sheep yogurt and cheese, or plain, unsweetened kefir (great in smoothies)

- Try making your own nut or seed milk (see recipe on modernmediterranean.com)
- If you are concerned about getting enough calcium, eat more non-dairy foods that are high in calcium, like cruciferous vegetables, nuts and seeds, beans, and bone-in fish

Healthy Hydration

An adult eliminates about 2–4 pints of water each day through urine, sweat, and breathing. You need to replenish at least the same volume through food and drink. This is particularly important for people undergoing chemotherapy, because a steady intake of water can help flush out chemo's toxic byproducts.

Although sodas, juices from concentrates, sweetened milk or yogurt beverages, and caffeinated drinks may contribute to hydration needs, they also contain sweeteners, colorings, flavorings, preservatives, caffeine, and, in the case of many soft drinks, bone-weakening carbonic and phosphoric acids. Avoid them whenever possible.

How Much?

The "8 x 8" rule—eight 8-ounce glasses of fluid—is an adequate starting point. A slightly more helpful guideline is to drink half your weight in fluid ounces (e.g., if you weigh 140 lbs, that's 70 ounces—or nearly 9 cups—of fluids). You'll need to drink even more under the following conditions:

- Exercise or any activity that makes you sweat (add an extra 1.5–2.5 cups of fluid; include electrolytes if you sweat heavily)
- Hot or humid weather
- Heated indoor air
- Altitude greater than 8,200 feet (2,500 meters)
- Fever, vomiting, or diarrhea
- Bladder infection or urinary tract stones
- Pregnancy or breastfeeding

If you're adequately hydrated, your urine should be pale yellow. Another good hydration yardstick is how often you go to the bathroom; when adequately hydrated, you should urinate about six to eight times in a 24-hour period.

Did you notice we're using the word "fluids," rather than water? Water is best, but it isn't the only substance that hydrates. All fluids—including soups, broths, teas, vegetables and fruits—count toward your fluid intake. The most hydrating foods include:

- 90–99% water content: cucumbers, cantaloupe, watermelon, lettuce, tomatoes, cabbage, celery, nonfat milk, spinach, summer squash, zucchini
- 80–89% water content: yogurt, apples, grapes, oranges, carrots, broccoli (cooked)
- 70–79% water content: bananas, avocados, cottage cheese, ricotta cheese, shrimp

If you're adequately hydrated, your urine should be pale yellow. Another good hydration yardstick is how often you go to the bathroom; when adequately hydrated, you should urinate every two to four hours during the day. (If you go significantly more often than that, check with your doctor.) Like daily bowel movements, healthy urination also helps your body eliminate toxins.

Hydration is particularly important for anyone experiencing diarrhea or vomiting, or who practices intermittent or prolonged fasting. Since all these factors can deplete the body's stores of electrolytes (sodium, potassium, magnesium, and calcium), we recommend that you add these to your water when fasting or experiencing digestive distress. You can buy sugar-free electrolyte powders (our favorite brands include ultimareplenisher.com or drinklmnt.com) or make your own electrolyte drink.

To make your own electrolyte drink (recipe from wellnessmama.com), fill a quart mason jar with:

- 1 quart liquid (such as freshly brewed green or herbal tea, coconut water, or plain water)

- 1/8–1/4 tsp Himalayan salt
- 1 tsp calcium-magnesium powder (available at naturalvitality.com)
- 1/4 cup or more 100% fruit juice (optional)
- a few drops of liquid stevia, a few spoonfuls of a non-glycemic sweetener like monk fruit or allulose, or a little honey or maple syrup (optional)

Mix or shake well. Cool and store for up to four days in refrigerator until ready to use.

Tea and Coffee

While most westerners drink black tea, people in Japan, China, and the north African rim of the Mediterranean prefer green and white tea.

All three come from the same plant, but white tea is the least processed and provides the largest quantity of antioxidant compounds, notably a flavonoid by the tongue-twisting name of epigallocatechin-3-gallate (EGCG). The green teas with the highest EGCG levels are the Japanese Sencha, Gyokuro, and Matcha teas, followed by Chinese Yunnan and Yuzan teas.

Green tea is thought to have significant cancer-protective effects, including inhibiting angiogenesis (see p. 186) and triggering the death of cancer cells. It may also reinforce the effects of certain chemotherapeutic agents while lessening their negative side effects.

Unfortunately, decaffeinated green tea contains only a third of the EGCG found in regular tea. To reduce caffeine but maintain optimal EGCG levels, infuse regular green tea for one to two minutes in hot water, pour off the liquid, add more hot water and steep for about eight minutes. Adding lemon juice to green tea helps to stabilize EGCG levels, which means you can drink it hours later, chilled, and still obtain good EGCG intake.

Contrary to popular belief, caffeinated beverages, including coffee, can contribute to your body's daily fluid requirement. Moderate coffee consumption does not lead to dehydration, and recent studies have found no connection between coffee and increased cancer risk. If anything, some studies associate coffee drinking with a *lower* risk of overall mortality.

Coffee is so high in antioxidants that the average person eating a typical Western diet gets more antioxidants from coffee than from consuming fruits, tea, red wine, cereal, and vegetables combined, because their consumption of the latter is so low. The polyphenols in coffee also support a healthy gut flora. Choose organic coffee if you can, as non-organic coffee is a crop that is heavily sprayed with pesticides.

Excessive coffee consumption, though, can cause problems. For one, the acid in coffee can contribute to acid reflux (try drinking low-acid coffee). Moreover, too much caffeine can lead to anxiety, heart palpitations, and panic attacks. If you're battling treatment-related fatigue, you may be tempted to boost energy levels with a strong cup of java, but be warned that caffeine can also disrupt sleep, which may make you feel even more tired the next day.

Red Wine

Red wine contains plant chemicals that are thought to lower the risk of heart disease, but that doesn't mean alcohol protects against cancer—on the contrary.

While compounds in red wine, such as resveratrol, anthocyanidins, and procyanidins, are powerful antioxidants, the ethanol in alcoholic drinks contributes to several common cancers, including those of the breast, mouth and throat, and esophagus; some research also links it to liver and bowel cancer. The risk of alcohol-related cancers is even greater in smokers.

The American Institute for Cancer Research is clear: For cancer prevention, it's best not to drink alcohol. If you drink alcohol at all, the AICR recommends to do so on rare occasions and limit it to two drinks in a day for men and one for women. "One drink" is the equivalent of half a pint

(250 ml) of normal strength beer or cider, 1 oz (25 ml) spirits, or 4 oz (125 ml) wine.

People with pancreatic or liver disease and women who have a family history of breast cancer should abstain from alcohol completely.

Over to You: Hydration Action Plan

- Drink a tall glass of water after every visit to the bathroom
- Place notes and water pitchers or bottles in highly visible places; take a sip every time you walk past
- Keep a bottle of your favorite unsweetened iced tea or coffee, lemon- or lime-flavored water, or kombucha in the fridge
- Make a quart of electrolyte drink and sip on it when fasting or experiencing diarrhea or vomiting
- If caffeine disturbs your sleep, avoid drinking caffeinated drinks in the afternoon and evening and stick to decaffeinated coffee or caffeine-free herbal teas—or go completely decaf
- Instead of drinking wine, get its healthy polyphenols from raw cocoa, apples (especially the Red Delicious, Granny Smith, and Reinette varieties), crabapples, cranberries (fresh or dried), raspberries, pomegranates and their juice, persimmons, raw nuts (especially walnuts, but also almonds and hazelnuts with skins), cinnamon, tea, and mulberries.

Make Every Calorie Count: Nutrient Density

To maximize the amount of nutrients you take in, eat foods that contain a large number of nutrients and are relatively low in calories. These foods are described as "nutrient dense."

The most nutrient-dense foods—highest in nutrients, lowest in calories—include:

- Berries
- Seaweed
- Mushrooms
- Garlic
- Fresh herbs and spices
- All leafy, green vegetables

You can eat as much of these foods as you want without overdoing calories. Of course, there are many other highly nutritious foods, such as avocados, nuts, oily fish, beans, fruits, liver, seafood, and meat, but these contain more calories, so pay attention to portion sizes.

In contrast, "energy-dense" foods are high in calories (energy) but low in nutrients. These empty-calorie foods often leave you with a nagging sense of dissatisfaction and cravings because your body is clamoring for *nutrients*, not just calories.

Examples of energy-dense, empty-calorie foods include:

- White breads and bagels
- Refined pasta, rice, and rice noodles
- Cakes and cookies
- Sweets and candy
- Ice cream
- Soft drinks and fruit-flavored beverages
- Margarine and shortening
- Store-bought salad dressings
- Frying fats and trans fats
- Alcoholic drinks

Use a tool such as the Nutrient Optimiser (nutrientoptimiser.com) to choose the most nutrient-dense foods, and use them to swap out empty-calorie choices.

Over to You: Nutrient Density Action Plan

- Every time you go to put food in your mouth, ask yourself: "Does this food contain nutrients?" If the food is made with processed ingredients (for instance, pasta made with white flour) or comes out of a package that lists more than five ingredients, it may not be very nutrient-dense. If you decide to eat it anyway, accompany it with vegetables, fish, herbs or other nutrient-dense foods.
- Track your diet on Cronometer and check the nutrient scores underneath the food diary; they'll tell you which nutrients you're missing and which foods provide them; adjust your diet accordingly
- Eat minimally processed foods, as these contain more nutrients than processed foods do
- Eat foods that are high in nutrients and low in calories, such as non-starchy vegetables, berries, seaweed, herbs, and spices

Vary the Foods You Eat

Dietary variety is a key element of a nutritious diet. That's because eating lots of *different* healthy foods increases your intake of essential nutrients, while simultaneously reducing the potential impact of overeating potentially damaging compounds that naturally occur in many foods.

Take beets: they contain contain healthy plant compounds called betalains that aren't found in any other food, so it's a great idea to eat them regularly. But if you ate beets every day, you might consume too much oxalic acid, a compound that increases your risk of kidney stones and makes it more difficult for your body to absorb calcium.

Nutrient Synergies

Research shows that eating a wide array of healthy foods lowers the risk of developing cancer. Eating various foods *within the same meal* is even better, because different nutrients eaten together can reinforce each other's cancer-fighting effects. This is called nutrition synergy.

For example, the antioxidant effect of lycopene, found particularly in tomatoes, is improved by other foods, such as green tea and omega-3 fats in fish. Eating healthy fats, such as avocados or nuts, with your vegetables helps your body absorb plants' protective phytochemicals.

Even people who are genetically predisposed to cancer appear to benefit from the synergistic effect of eating a wide variety of plant foods. At the University of Montreal, a team of scientists studied women who carry the BRCA1 and BRCA2 genes associated with a significantly elevated risk of developing breast cancer and ovarian cancer. The greater the variety of fruits and vegetables these women ate, the less risk they had of developing cancer. Those who ate more than 23 *different* fruits and vegetables per week reduced their cancer risk by 73% compared to those who ate the least varied produce.

Examples of synergistic food combinations:

- Mixed salad with three types of greens (such as romaine lettuce, arugula, radicchio), sliced red onion, apple cubes, walnuts, grapes, blue cheese, grated carrot, and a dressing of olive oil and lemon juice
- Chicken stew with onion, garlic, celery, carrots, mushrooms, leek, potato, thyme, parsley, bay leaf, red wine, and olive oil
- Minestrone made from onions, garlic, peppers, tomatoes, thyme, bay leaf, olive oil, and beans, drizzled with basil pesto

- A stir-fry of onions, ginger, garlic, red bell pepper, yellow bell pepper, eggplant, mushrooms, cilantro, and a little brown rice cooked in olive and sesame oil
- Freshly pressed juice of carrots, apple, celery, and ginger with a smidgen of olive oil

Eat Seasonally

One of the easiest ways to ensure dietary diversity and nutrient synergies is to adapt your diet to the changing seasons. What's in season in May won't be the same as in October, so your meals will undergo a constant rotation.

The table below lists the seasonal vegetables and fruits available in the northern hemisphere. Don't use the store's produce aisle as your guide; most supermarkets stock out-of-season items, which won't be as tasty or nutritious as in-season choices. The table below lists the seasonal vegetables and fruits available in the northern hemisphere. Vary your produce in time with the changing seasons.

Table 1: Eat with the Seasons

Spring	**Summer**	**Fall (Autumn)**	**Winter**
Fresh, green, tender, eaten raw or lightly cooked	Light, cooling, moist, mostly eaten raw	More warming foods and spices, mostly eaten cooked	Warming foods and spices, usually cooked
Asparagus Avocados Basil Beans Beets Berries Broccoli Cabbage (green, white, cauliflower) Green/spring onions Leafy greens (like chard, collard greens, kale, mustard greens, spinach) Lettuce Parsley Peas Radish Rhubarb Shallots Swiss chard Spinach Summer squash	Apricots Basil Beans Beets Berries Broccoli Cherries Cilantro Corn Cucumber Dates Eggplant Figs Garlic Grapes Leafy greens (like chard, collard greens, kale, mustard greens, spinach) Melons Peas Peaches Peppermint Peppers (spicy or sweet) Plums Summer Squash (e.g. zucchini, marrow) Tomatoes Watermelon	Apples Broccoli Brussels sprouts Cabbage (red, cauliflower, Chinese, etc.) Celery (root and stalks) Cranberries Cucumber Dates Endives Fennel Grapes Leafy greens (like chard, collard greens, kale, mustard greens, spinach) Lettuce Mushrooms Nuts Mandarins Pears Peppers Persimmons Pomegranates Quinces Root vegetables (carrots, parsnips, etc.) Shallots Sweet potatoes Onions	Avocados Broccoli Cabbage (red, kale, savoy, cauliflower, Brussels sprouts, etc.) Celery (root and stalks) Chicory Fennel Grapefruit Leafy greens (like chard, collard greens, kale, mustard greens, spinach) Wild mushrooms Mandarin oranges Onions Pears Root vegetables (like carrots, parsnips, beets, potatoes) Sweet potatoes Warming seasonings (like ginger, pepper, mustard)

Modern food processing methods have made it possible to freeze produce and eat it throughout the year, or to obtain vegetables grown in hothouses outside their natural growing season. So, while local seasonal produce is best, go ahead and enjoy berries, bell peppers, or zucchini in winter occasionally. It's always better to eat an out-of-season vegetable or fruit than to not eat any at all.

Over to You: Nutrient Synergy and Dietary Diversity Action Plan

- Try to eat vegetables and fruits of different colors—for instance, alternate between red and green apples; white and red onions; green and red cabbage; white, brown, and black beans, etc.; a food's colors reflect its individual nutritional profile, so varying colors means broadening the range of nutrients you eat
- Each time you serve yourself food, look at your plate and identify the different colors on it; try get at least three different colors into any dish
- Plan meals ahead of time; with a plan, you can intentionally vary your proteins (meat, fish, dairy, eggs), your produce, your grains, your beans, etc.
- Learn new recipes; use magazines and videos, attend cooking classes, or sign up for a healthy meal-kit delivery service to give you some fresh ideas for tasty, healthy meals; get recipes from modernmediterranean.com
- Subscribe to a community-supported agriculture (CSA) program where you'll receive a selection of produce every week that changes with the seasons

Organic or Conventional?

The use of manmade pesticides, herbicides, and fungicides in crop farming has increased sharply in the past few decades. The most heavily used agricultural pesticide is glyphosate, classified by the World Health Organization's International Agency for Research on Cancer (IARC) as "probably carcinogenic to humans."

In 2018, more than half of the 10,545 fresh and processed food samples tested by the USDA had detectable pesticide residues; 21% of the samples contained one pesticide, and 31.2% had more than one pesticide. Even though less than 1% of the samples had levels above legal limits, this is nonetheless a disappointing finding, given rising consumer demand for food without agrochemical residues.

While there is some controversy around the effects of agricultural toxins in foods, it's known that direct exposure to pesticides around the home and in agriculture increases the risk of cancer.

The Dirty Dozen and Clean Fifteen

Since fruits and vegetables account for most pesticide residues in the diet, it's important to know which are the most affected.

The Environmental Working Group (EWG) publishes an annual shopper's guide (see ewg.org/foodnews/dirty-dozen.php) highlighting the most contaminated ("Dirty Dozen") and the least contaminated ("Clean Fifteen") produce.

Table 2: Most and Least Contaminated Produce, 2021

Vegetables – most pesticide residues	Fruits – most pesticide residues	Vegetables – least pesticide residues	Fruits – least pesticide residues
Spinach	Strawberries	Sweet corn	Avocados
Kale, collard and mustard greens	Nectarines	Onions	Pineapple
Bell and hot peppers	Apples	Sweet peas	Papaya
Celery	Grapes	Eggplant	Kiwi
Tomatoes	Cherries	Asparagus	Honeydew melon
Potatoes	Peaches	Broccoli	Cantaloupe
Cherry tomatoes	Pears	Cabbage	Mangoes
Lettuce	Blueberries	Cauliflower	Watermelon
Cucumbers	Plums	Mushrooms	Bananas
Green beans	Tangerines	Sweet potatoes	Oranges
	Grapefruit	Winter and summer squashes	Raspberries

You don't have to memorize these lists: Just install the EWG's Healthy Living app on your smartphone and consult it when you go shopping. Or consult the Dirty Dozen/Clean Fifteen lists on the EWG's website, using the web link above.

Keep in mind that fresh fruits and vegetables are among the best sources of natural cancer-protective compounds, and the benefits of eating them—even non-organic—outweigh the possible side effects of pesticide residues. Using the EWG findings can help you minimize potential pesticide exposure.

Eat Well Without Breaking the Bank

The cost of organic food doesn't have to be prohibitive. Here are tips ways to eat nutritious and mostly organic food, without exploding your food budget.

- **Be selective.** If there are foods that you eat frequently or that carry high pesticide residues ("Dirty Dozen"), replace these with organic equivalents. Foods with low exposures ("Clean Fifteen") can be non-organic.

- **Shop creatively.** Find alternative sources of low-residue foods, such as farmers' markets and health food co-ops. You can also order organic food—mostly dried staples like beans, rice, grains, or dried fruit—online. We like the organic online co-op Thrive Market (thrivemarket.com), where organic foods and body- and home-care products cost around 20–40% less than in regular stores.
- **Shop in bulk.** It's often more cost-effective to buy dry organic goods from self-service bins rather than in sealed packages. Buying a whole tray of organic peaches or zucchini is often less expensive than buying them individually weighed. Large bags of organic frozen vegetables and fruits often cost less than smaller portions, and since they are frozen, you can use as much as you need and return the rest to the freezer for later.
- **Shop seasonally and locally.** Out-of-season fruits and vegetables are often expensively transported over long distances. Locally grown seasonal produce is cheaper—and better for the environment.
- **Subscribe to a Community Supported Agriculture program:** CSA schemes cut out the middleman and provide fresh, locally grown—and sometimes organic—produce straight to consumers, usually at a lower cost than at the grocery store. You can find a CSA near you by consulting the US Department of Agriculture's CSA directory: ams.usda.gov/local-food-directories/csas. If you want affordable organic vegetables delivered to your home, check out services that deliver "ugly" organic produce (i.e., not pretty enough for supermarkets) directly to consumers. Examples include misfitsmarket.com and hungryharvest.net.
- **Buy house brands.** Since any food with the word "organic" on its label has to go through the same USDA-Certified process, save money by buying store-branded organic products.

- **Eat meat sparingly.** Most people don't need more than 3–4 oz of meat (the size of a deck of cards) per meal. You can save money by buying organic meat and eggs directly from producers rather than from supermarkets. Some meat producers ship directly to consumers (North American directory of farms that ship direct to consumers: eatwild.com/products/farmsthatship.html). Stretch what you buy by replacing some of the meat with cooked lentils, which add flavor, fiber, and plant nutrients. And buy cheaper cuts: stewing beef, oxtail, beef cheeks, and organ meats such as liver, tongue, and gizzards are inexpensive, highly nutritious, and tasty.
- **Plan meals.** Plan your meals around your budget, make a shopping list, and stick to it to avoid impulse purchases. Buy only what you need. Freeze or recycle any leftovers into another dish.
- **D.I.Y.** Instead of buying expensive pre-washed, pre-chopped vegetables or fruits, get them whole, wash and chop them yourself, and pack them into containers or sealable plastic bags to refrigerate or freeze.
- **Avoid processed organics.** While organic sodas, pretzels, or cookies may appear healthier, they're still packed with sugar, sodium, and white flour, and devoid of nutrition. Junk is junk, no matter how "organic."

Clean produce thoroughly. If you can't afford or obtain organic produce, here are some ways to reduce your exposure to pesticide residues on foods:

- Wash fruits and vegetables (including organic) under running water for 30–60 seconds; rub gently to dislodge residues
- Scrub edible skins (apples, pears) with a clean produce brush; wash brushes regularly with hot soapy water or in a dishwasher; dry completely
- Bicarbonate wash: Researchers at the University of Massachusetts Amherst have discovered that soaking produce in a mixture of baking soda and water removes

pesticide residues: mix one teaspoon of baking soda with two cups of water and submerge produce for two minutes or more (the longer you soak, the more chemicals you get rid of); rinse in tap water again before eating
- Wash inedible skins (bananas, oranges) before removing to prevent contamination on your hands and on the edible parts
- Remove outer leaves of heads of lettuce or cabbages—that's where most pesticide residues are
- If you use citrus peel (such as zest), buy organic.

Over to You: Organic Food Action Plan

- Study the Dirty Dozen and Clean Fifteen lists and adjust your shopping habits where needed. For instance, if you frequently eat spinach or strawberries, find organic versions of these; if they're too expensive fresh, get frozen organic spinach and berries
- Explore farmers' markets, farm stores and co-ops near you; study their special offers
- Explore online stores that deliver organic food, both fresh, frozen, and dried; share a co-op membership with a friend or neighbor to reduce subscription costs
- If you have a garden, consider growing some delicious organic produce; the book *Eating on the Wild Side* by Jo Robinson is an invaluable guide for anyone wishing to grow nutrient-dense vegetables and fruits

Can You Treat Cancer With Nutrition?

On the topic of "anticancer" diets—eating plans that claim to cure cancer—there's good news and bad news.

On the plus side, each of these diets—be it alkaline, macrobiotic, vegan, or keto—includes beneficial elements. But here's the bad news: diet alone has never been scientifically proven to cure cancer, and when it replaces or delays more effective treatments and weakens the body, a special "anticancer" diet may even be harmful.

The American Cancer Society (ACS) and the American Institute for Cancer Research (AICR) have dietary guidelines for cancer patients that emphasize plant-rich, nutrient-dense eating patterns (see appendix for links). These are very general and should be adapted to each individual, ideally in consultation with a nutrition professional.

Studies suggest that a high level of adherence to the ACS and AICR guidelines decreases the risk of developing cancer by 17% to over 50% (depending on cancer site) and decreases cancer-specific mortality by 20–30%. And yet, cancer patients and survivors rarely follow these guidelines. Instead, as many as 48% of cancer patients adopt "special diets" that are based on little or no scientific evidence.

In 2014 a team of German researchers simulated an internet search a cancer patient might conduct, using the search term "cancer diet." The diets that came up most frequently included alkaline diets, raw-food diets, macrobiotics, the Gerson diet, the Budwig diet, and low-carbohydrate or ketogenic diets. After examining these diets' anti-cancer credentials, they concluded: "We did not find clinical evidence supporting any of the diets. Furthermore, case reports and pre-clinical data point to the potential harm of some of these diets" (see pubmed.ncbi.nlm.nih.gov/24403443).

Four years later, an American team of cancer researchers published their analysis of "anticancer" diets in the journal *Oncology* (see pubmed.ncbi.nlm.nih.gov/30474102). While they highlighted various benefits of the diets they studied (alkaline, low-carb/keto, paleo, macrobiotic, and vegan), they also listed their negative aspects, notably: "[P]seudo-scientific rationales for their anti-cancer properties, limited evidence that they improve cancer outcomes, the possibility for nutrient insufficiencies, and elimination of food groups proven beneficial for cancer prevention and general health."

Another potential risk of "anticancer" diets is that they can cause people to develop a highly restrictive—even obsessive—mindset around food, which can be stressful. In some cases, this can lead to orthorexia, a medical condition in which the sufferer systematically avoids specific foods in the belief that they are harmful, which can lead to unintended weight loss and nutritional deficiencies.

Let's look at the "anticancer" diets we are most frequently asked about (in alphabetical order):

Alkaline diet

You've probably read on the internet that cancer cells only grow in acidic environments, which is why you should eat an alkalizing diet. Promoters of the alkaline diet theory believe that eating certain foods—such as meat, fish, dairy, and grains—makes your body "acidic" and promotes the development of cancer, whereas foods like vegetables and fruits make the body "alkaline" and reduce cancer risk.

Alas, to date, no scientific inquiry has discovered a clear link between the acidity or alkalinity of people's diets and their risk of developing cancer. We do know that plant-rich diets are associated with a reduced risk of cancer and cancer-related death, while diets that are heavy in refined grains and animal products are more often associated with increased cancer risks. However, the health benefits of fruits and vegetables are probably due to other factors than how acidic or alkaline they make your body.

For one, the only two studies that have investigated the association of dietary acid load with cancer did not yield conclusive results.

Moreover, the alkaline theory rests on the flawed assumption that cancers need acidic environments to grow. In fact, cancer can grow quite happily in alkaline tissue; indeed, in many test tube experiments, cancer cells are grown in an environment at a slightly alkaline pH of 7.4.

We know that the immediate environment around cancer cells is often acidic. It is not, however, the acidic environment that promotes the growth of the tumor but, conversely, the tumor that creates the acidic environment through the way it makes energy and uses oxygen. Once a tumor is established, blood pH in the surrounding tissues is unlikely to have any effect on the pH of the cancer.

Having said all this, we encourage you to eat plenty of plant foods anyway; they not only support a healthy intestinal flora but also contain nutrients that reduce your risk of developing and dying from cancer and other chronic diseases. Therefore, boosting your intake of vegetables and fruits, and reducing consumption of sugar and refined grains—in other words: eating a nutrient-dense diet—is a good idea, regardless of its effect on your acid–alkaline balance.

Gerson Therapy

The Gerson therapy is an alternative cancer treatment involving coffee enemas, supplements, juicing, and a special diet that is claimed to cleanse the body, boost the immune system, and stimulate metabolism.

The Gerson therapy requires following a strict low-salt, low-fat, vegetarian diet and drinking the freshly pressed juice of about 20 lbs of fresh fruits and vegetables each day. In addition, patients must take up to five coffee enemas each day. Various supplements, such as potassium, vitamin B12, pancreatic enzymes, thyroid hormone, and a special iodine solution are used. All of this is intended to stimulate organ function, particularly of the liver and thyroid.

There is scant proof of the efficacy of the Gerson diet, however. What research has been produced by Gerson diet proponents has been plagued by flawed methodologies, small sample sizes, inconclusive results, and other problems (such as a large percentage of patients not completing the study), making it impossible to draw clear conclusions about the effectiveness of treatment.

Some aspects of the Gerson regimen, such as eating or drinking fruits and vegetables, can be part of a healthy diet. However, eating such an imbalanced diet, especially over an extended period of time, can be deleterious to people who are already ill and weakened by cancer treatments. Moreover, a high intake of juiced fruits and carrots might cause elevated glucose and insulin levels.

There is precious little scientific evidence to support some of the other components of the Gerson diet, such as consuming only fresh, raw juices prepared in a certain way, eliminating salt from the diet, minimizing fat and protein intake, and taking coffee enemas and liver extract injections. Due to a lack of research, not much is known about the safety of the Gerson diet. Patients undergoing the Gerson therapy may experience a number of adverse effects, including dizziness and weakness, abdominal cramps, loss of appetite, diarrhea and sickness, cold sores, aching, fever, and sweating. Coffee enemas may result in electrolyte imbalance, which could in turn cause infection, dehydration, colitis, constipation, heart and lung problems, and even death.

Ketogenic Diet

A ketogenic, or "keto," diet is one that replaces the body's typical go-to energy source—carbohydrates—with fats. When you eat a keto diet, you derive 70–80% of your calories from fat, while carbohydrate intake is restricted to 20–30 g a day. This macronutrient composition forces the body to burn fat rather than carbohydrate, shifting the body's primary fuel from glucose to ketones (the byproduct of fat burning).

Keto diets allow fish, meat, eggs, dairy, nuts, seeds, fats, and oils, but exclude foods that are high in carbohydrate, such as pasta, bread, rice and other grain-based foods, potatoes, legumes, and most fruits. Non-starchy vegetables like leafy greens and small servings of low-sugar fruits like berries are usually permitted.

It has been known for the last 100 years that cancer cells rely heavily on glucose for energy. Epidemiological studies show that chronically elevated blood glucose levels—for instance in people with diabetes—are associated with increased risk of cancer. Moreover, in molecular models, high levels of glucose are associated with increased cancer growth, while depriving cancer cells of glucose appears to prompt apoptosis (cancer cell suicide).

Because glucose is derived primarily from carbohydrates, it's thought that by minimizing carbohydrate intake, you can lower glucose, insulin, and IGF-1 levels (see p. 104) and thereby starve cancer cells. Indeed, the ketogenic diet has been shown to improve cancer outcomes in patients with aggressive glioma brain tumors and may be effective against cancers that take up sugar on PET/CT scans. However, glucose restriction doesn't always work; some tumor cells are able to use ketones for energy.

Ketogenic diets may have additional cancer-fighting mechanisms. For instance, they can induce oxidative stress in cancer cells, thereby reinforcing the effect of chemotherapy and radiation. Ketogenic diets may also help preserve muscle tissue in people with cachexia. And in animal models, ketogenic diets have been shown to decrease the initiation, progression, and metastasis of cancer.

While the keto diet certainly looks promising, rigorous scientific evidence for its cancer-therapeutic benefits is limited. Small human studies suggest that ketogenic diets are safe and do not have a negative impact on quality of life; that's a good start. However, it's not yet clear how far-reaching their benefits are.

As the authors of "Pros and Cons of Dietary Strategies Popular Among Cancer Patients" write in their Nov. 15, 2018, article in *Oncology*, "Ketogenic diets may have utility in certain individuals, especially in combination with other conventional therapies, but there is currently no reliable way to predict which patients might respond."

Furthermore, keto diets can be difficult to implement without expert dietary counseling, and a poorly formulated ketogenic diet (sometimes described as "dirty keto") could incur nutrient deficiencies. Moreover, because of the restrictive nature of keto diets, sharing meals with friends and family and eating out can be difficult.

So, while a ketogenic diet may provide powerful therapeutic support to people in cancer treatment, slightly higher carb intakes (50–100 g net carbs a day) may be an effective long-term maintenance strategy to keep glucose and insulin levels low without incurring the risk of nutritional deficiencies or dieting burnout.

If you are interested in trying a keto diet, discuss this with your doctor first. If your doctor OKs this approach, we recommend that you eat a Mediterranean keto diet that contains plenty of oily fish, plant fats, and anti-inflammatory vegetables, herbs, and spices. To help you transition to this way of eating, work with a reputable nutrition professional who has a deep expertise in this area, rather than relying on meal plans and cookbooks sold online by keto enthusiasts. See the Resources section for keto books and websites we recommend.

Macrobiotic Diet

Macrobiotics encompass a philosophy, a cultural movement, and an eating pattern that is based in large part on the Eastern philosophical principles of yin and yang.

The typical macrobiotic diet is predominantly vegetarian and emphasizes unprocessed, organic foods. The diet, by weight, is up to 60% whole grains, 20–30% vegetables, and 5–10% legumes. Sea vegetables are cooked with the beans or as separate dishes. Fruits, white fish, and seeds and nuts can be consumed a few times per week or less often.

Dairy, eggs, coffee, sugar, aromatic herbs, red meat, poultry, and processed foods are discouraged. Some vegetables, such as potatoes, tomatoes, eggplant, peppers, asparagus, spinach, beets, zucchini, and avocados, are also discouraged. The diet also advises against eating fruit that does not grow locally.

We endorse many aspects of the macrobiotic diet, notably its emphasis on unprocessed foods, vegetables, legumes, intact grains and fiber, natural cookware, and mindful cooking and eating. However, unless great care is taken, the diet can be monotonous and imbalanced, and may contain too much carbohydrate relative to fat and protein. It may also be hard to obtain adequate amounts of vitamin B12, calcium, and vitamin D on a macrobiotic diet.

There are no research studies on the macrobiotic diet in cancer patients; however, we await with interest the results of DIANA (Diet and Androgens)-5, an ongoing randomized clinical trial in 1,208 breast cancer survivors investigating the effect of exercise and a Mediterranean-macrobiotic diet plan on weight loss and cancer recurrence (see pubmed.ncbi.nlm.nih.gov/22495696).

Raw Food Diet

While the internet teems with stories about people who claim to have healed their cancers by eating only raw foods, there is no scientific evidence that raw-food diets are effective at treating cancer.

The idea behind raw diets is that heating food destroys its nutrients and natural enzymes, which are thought to support digestion and fight disease. Some raw-foodists consume raw meat, fish, or milk, but, mostly, "raw-food diets" refer to vegan diets.

A typical raw vegan diet consists of raw foods only, and excludes processed foods as well as foods that are considered inedible raw, like dry beans, grains, and potatoes. Salt, vinegar, alcohol, and caffeine (coffee, tea) are also off-limits. Even stricter versions of the diet exclude oils, natural sweeteners (including honey and maple syrup), dried or dehydrated foods, onions, garlic, hot peppers, spices, and supplements.

Adherents of this type of diet must be disciplined and willing to spend a considerable amount of time in the kitchen to ensure their diet is varied and balanced enough to prevent nutritional deficiencies. Indeed, long-term followers of raw vegan diets risk experiencing deficiencies in iodine, calcium, vitamin B12, vitamin B2, vitamin D, and zinc.

To be sure, there is some evidence that raw food is more nutritious than cooked food. Cooking vegetables, for instance, decreases their water-soluble and heat-sensitive nutrients, such as carotenoids and vitamin C. The insoluble fiber in vegetables, which speeds up intestinal transit and promotes the excretion of carcinogens, also decreases as a result of cooking. Moreover, soil-based organisms on raw vegetables and fruits, which support our digestive and immune systems, are also destroyed by cooking.

Cooking can also create byproducts that may be harmful. In foods that are high in carbohydrates or protein, heat causes the so-called Maillard reaction, which denatures many essential amino acids and makes the food harder to digest. High-temperature food processing—particularly meat, dairy, grains, sugar, and some vegetable products—can also form inflammatory compounds called advanced glycation end-products (AGEs). And cooking meat at high temperatures or over open flames creates so-called heterocyclic amines (HCAs), which can cause cancer in animals, and polycyclic aromatic hydrocarbons (PAH), a known carcinogen in humans.

Having said all this, cooking also has health benefits. Heating vegetables increases the bioavailability of some carotenoids in certain vegetables, such as spinach, tomatoes, and carrots. Very importantly for people with weakened immune and digestive systems, cooking kills pathogenic microbes and makes food easier to digest and absorb.

Cooking also reduces natural compounds present in many foods that can cause health problems in humans, such as thyroid-disrupting goitrogens (found in cruciferous vegetables such as cabbage, broccoli, Brussels sprouts, cauliflower, bok choy, kale, and collard greens, as well as in soy and sweet potatoes), oxalic acid (a compound in spinach, chard, and beet greens that can interfere with calcium absorption and increase your risk of kidney stones), phytic acid (a.k.a. phytate, a compound found in whole grains, nuts, and seeds that can hinder the absorption of essential nutrients such as magnesium, calcium, zinc, and iron), and lectins, (carbohydrate-binding proteins found in many foods, especially legumes and grains, that can cause digestive problems).

Raw foods are an important part of a healthy diet and we are keen promoters of fresh, uncooked and fermented vegetables, fruits, salads and smoothies teeming with live, beneficial bacteria. However, there are times when cooked foods are more appropriate. Ideally, eat some of each.

Let's take our cues from traditional dietary patterns. In the Mediterranean, for example, summer is a time when vegetables are mostly eaten raw, in salads and sauces, as toppings and garnishes, or as cool, fresh soups (think Spanish gazpacho). During winter, on the other hand, foods are generally cooked and warming (think: pot au feu, a slowly simmered French beef and vegetable stew, and the many delicious Greek, Italian, and North African stews made from vegetables, dried beans, and grains).

Veg(etari)an Diets

Many people adopt vegetarian and vegan diets (which we will collectively describe here as "veg(etari)an") to fight or prevent cancer.

As you've probably figured by now, we're both huge fans of plant foods. However, while a well-planned veg(etari)an diet can be nutritious, we don't believe you need to cut out all animal products to lower your cancer risk. Indeed, many animal foods contain valuable nutrients, and eliminating them completely might cause deficiencies that undermine your health.

There's surprisingly little data to support the assumption that veg(etari)an diets are cancer-protective. Observational studies (a notoriously unreliable way of analyzing foods' effects on health) indicate that veg(etari)an diets offer modest protection: in a large meta-analysis published in 2017, vegetarian and vegan diets were associated with a reduced risk of developing cancer (of 8% and 15%, respectively) but no reduction in mortality—the risk of dying prematurely.

Also, several small randomized clinical trials in men with low-risk prostate cancer showed benefits of a low-fat vegan diet; however, this diet was delivered along with nutritional supplements, exercise, stress reduction, and social support interventions, making it hard to determine how much the diet itself contributed to the positive results.

Even where studies do show reduced cancer risk in veg(etari)ans, this may be due in part to the fact that people who eat veg(etari)an diets often have other healthy habits. For instance, veg(etari)ans are less likely to smoke or drink heavily and are more likely to eat fruits and vegetables, exercise, and have a normal body weight than non-veg(etari)ans. Although researchers try to adjust for these factors in their statistical analyses, the overall lifestyle of people who follow veg(etari)an diets may be reflected in the health benefits seen.

Interestingly, several studies investigating the mortality risk (from all causes, not just cancer) of vegetarians and health-conscious omnivores have found no difference between these two groups (both outlive the folks eating a standard American diet). Maybe non-dietary factors play a more important role than whether they eat meat or not?

If you're eating a standard American diet high in processed foods, refined grains, sugar, poor-quality meat, and unhealthy fats, shifting to a veg(etari)an diet would undoubtedly bring about noticeable improvements in your health and well-being. However, if all you do is omit animal foods without replacing them with nutritious plant-based equivalents, you run the risk of incurring nutritional imbalances over time. Indeed, veg(etari)an diets can lead to deficiencies in B12, certain amino acids, calcium, iron, zinc, the omega-3 fatty acids EPA and DHA, and fat-soluble vitamins like A and D.

Rather than restrict animal foods altogether, therefore, we recommend an omnivorous diet that's heavily plant-based but also contains small servings of carefully selected and prepared animal foods such as fish, meat, eggs, and dairy. This could be the Mediterranean diet or any other nutrient-dense diet that eschews processed food and prioritizes real, fresh, whole food.

If you eat a veg(etari)an diet for ethical or religious reasons, make sure it's as nutrient-dense as possible. This may require some research, meal planning, and a willingness to cook. If you are open to eating a wide variety of vegetables and fruits, legumes, seeds, nuts, and whole grains, and are willing to take nutritional supplements to obtain the nutrients that are hard to derive from plant foods, you can be very healthy on a veg(etari)an diet. We recommend you consult a nutritional professional to make sure you're getting all the nutrients you need.

In closing, before you undertake significant dietary changes—be they keto, veg(etari)an, raw-food, etc.—talk to your cancer care team or to an experienced nutrition expert. Research the diet in reputable medical journals and find out all you can about outcomes and side effects.

Chapter 4

Boost Your Body's Defense Systems

In the previous section we looked at ways in which your diet can help create a biological environment that's inhospitable to cancer cells. Our bodies don't solely depend on external inputs like food to resist cancer; the body has many powerful mechanisms of its own that can counter the development and spread of tumors. This section takes a closer look at these.

Fighting Oxidation and Inflammation

Oxidation and inflammation are closely connected chemical reactions in the body. Within limits, both are normal, healthy processes, but if allowed to get out of hand, they can pave the way for health problems, including cancer.

Oxidation

Excess oxygen results in the creation of so-called reactive oxygen species, known as free radicals. Free radicals damage cells' fatty cell membranes, proteins, and DNA and lead to faulty cell replication.

Some free radicals arise from the body's normal metabolic functions, such as converting food into energy (metabolism), exercising, and fighting bacterial, viral, or fungal infections. External factors, such as pollution, chemical toxins, radiation (including excessive sunbathing), cigarette smoke, pesticides, stress, lack of sleep, high blood sugar levels, high intakes of polyunsaturated fatty acids, excessive intake of iron, magnesium, copper, or zinc, and a sedentary lifestyle also create free radicals. Food sources of free radicals include burned, barbecued, or smoked foods and rancid fats.

Thankfully, antioxidants—compounds that neutralize free radicals—can be produced by the body or obtained through foods. Antioxidants produced in the body include superoxide dismutase, alpha lipoic acid, and glutathione. Antioxidant nutrients include vitamins A, C, E, the members of the carotene family, the minerals selenium, copper, zinc, and manganese, and a variety of other plant chemicals. All of these compounds are particularly prevalent in plant foods, and they work best as a team.

When oxidative stress exceeds the protective antioxidant defense shield, the result is chronic inflammation.

Inflammation

Inflammation is the body's response to trauma. While this is a good thing when dealing with acute injuries, frequent or chronic inflammation can trigger the production of cancer cells and sustain their growth and spread.

After a cancer diagnosis, it's important to keep chronic, low-level inflammation as low as possible, because it can lead to:

- Increased cancer growth rates
- Increased cancer spread (metastases)
- Increased resistance to cancer treatments
- Increased cancer recurrence rates
- Increased rates of dying from cancer
- Increased pain and fatigue
- Decreased appetite and increased muscle loss (cachexia)

You can tame chronic, low-level inflammation by:

- Getting adequate amounts of aerobic exercise (p. 193)
- Getting adequate amounts of sleep (p. 213)
- Eliminating pollutants like tobacco (p. 226)

- Addressing low-level, constant irritation, such as acid reflux
- Practicing stress reduction (p. 243)
- Losing excess body fat (especially around the belly) and increasing muscle mass
- Correcting nutrient deficiencies, especially vitamins A, B12, C, folic acid, iron, selenium, and zinc
- Supporting healthy gut microbes (p. 179)
- Taking COX-2 inhibitors (ask your doctor first)
- Taking anti-inflammatory supplements (ask your doctor first), such as alpha-lipoic acid (ALA), ashwagandha, barley grass, boswellia, digestive enzymes, omega-3 fatty acids (EPA and DHA), quercetin or rutin, resveratrol, and selenium

One of the most important steps you can take is to adopt an anti-inflammatory diet. This means avoiding:

- Processed oils high in omega-6 fatty acids (e.g., soybean, corn, safflower, sunflower, and cottonseed oils)
- Trans fats
- Added sugar
- Refined grains—anything made with wheat flour, other refined starches (such as tapioca, corn, potato, etc.), as well as white rice, rice flour, rice noodles or rice cakes
- Synthetic food additives
- Alcohol
- Charred or barbecued meat
- Fried food
- Any foods you are allergic or sensitive to

And it means eating more:

- Antioxidant-rich plant foods
- Brightly colored fruits (especially berries) and vegetables
- Nuts and seeds
- Legumes
- Garlic and onions

- Omega-3-rich foods, such as salmon, sardines, and mackerel
- Antioxidant nutrients: vitamins A, C, E, niacin, CoQ10, and members of the carotene family
- Antioxidant minerals: selenium, copper, zinc, and manganese
- Fresh and dried cooking herbs: ginger (freshly grated is more potent than dried), turmeric, curry, cinnamon, cayenne pepper, black pepper, oregano, basil, chives, cilantro, and cumin
- Teas: green, goldenseal, calendula, echinacea

Aspirin and NSAIDs

Do you regularly take an aspirin or NSAID (non-steroidal anti-inflammatory drug) for aches and pains or heart-disease prevention? If so, you might also be protecting yourself from cancer.

Aspirin has many anticancer effects, including encouraging precancerous or cancerous cell death, calming inflammation, inhibiting the growth of new blood vessels to nourish a growing tumor (angiogenesis; see p. 186), and other proposed mechanisms.

An analysis of various studies found that it takes about five years before any anticancer benefit of aspirin appears. That said, taking a daily baby aspirin (an NSAID) has also shown increased survival in various cancers:

- **Breast cancer:** A 2011 study showed that women who took aspirin had a roughly 20% lower risk of breast cancer than non-users (pubmed.ncbi.nlm.nih.gov/20669045). In another study, breast cancer survivors who took a daily aspirin were 43% less likely to have recurrence and 64% less likely to die from the disease (pubmed.ncbi.nlm.nih.gov/20159825).
- **Ovarian cancer:** In a study of 20,000 women, those who used aspirin daily had a 20% lower risk of ovarian

cancer than those who used aspirin less than once a week (pubmed.ncbi.nlm.nih.gov/24503200).

- **Colorectal cancer:** One large study found that taking 75 mg aspirin (similar to the amount in a "baby" or low-dose aspirin) for five or more years decreased the risk of colon cancer by up to 70% and lowered the risk of developing rectal cancer by 40% (pubmed.ncbi.nlm.nih.gov/20970847).
- **Melanoma:** In a study of nearly 60,000 women, those who used aspirin had a 21% lower risk of melanoma compared with non-users. The longer the women used aspirin, the lower their risk (pubmed.ncbi.nlm.nih.gov/23483536).
- **Prostate cancer:** In a study of 5,955 men who received surgery or radiation therapy for prostate cancer, those who regularly used aspirin (any dose) had a 57% lower risk of dying from prostate cancer than non-users, a lower risk of recurrence, and a lower risk of developing bone metastases (pubmed.ncbi.nlm.nih.gov/22927523).
- **Metastasis (cancer spread):** In one meta-analysis, in which investigators identified 987 new cancer (solid tumors) diagnoses, aspirin use reduced the risk of being diagnosed with a metastasized cancer by 18–46% (pubmed.ncbi.nlm.nih.gov/22440947).

Still, studies are mixed. One meta-analysis of over 100,000 patients followed for five years found that aspirin use did not significantly reduce risk of cancer-related mortality or incidence—possibly because the duration of aspirin use was not long enough.

It should be noted that NSAIDs like aspirin can increase bleeding risk, reduce the effectiveness of other medications, cause gastrointestinal side effects, and pose risk to the kidneys. For most healthy people, however, the risks of taking a daily, low-dose aspirin (75–81 mg) are nominal and the potential anticancer benefits are significant. If you're not currently taking a daily, low-dose aspirin, discuss the potential risks and benefits with your healthcare team.

Over to You: Your Antioxidant, Anti-Inflammatory Action Plan

- Assess your exposure to factors that cause oxidation and inflammation; reduce these, one by one. If this feels overwhelming, enlist the support of a friend or coach.
- Eat antioxidant and anti-inflammatory foods at every meal; introduce these, one by one. If this feels overwhelming, work with a nutritionist or dietitian.
- Ask your doctor whether taking aspirin daily is safe and appropriate for you.

Feed Your Immune System

In the rapidly advancing field of cancer immunology, researchers are developing new therapies that either stimulate the immune system or counteract immune-suppressing responses.

To date, immune therapies include:

- Monoclonal antibodies that attack a specific part of a cancer cell
- CAR T-cell therapy: taking T-cells from the patient, changing them to recognize cancer cells, and reinjecting them back into the patient
- Immune checkpoint inhibitors that help the immune system recognize cancer cells and mount an attack
- Vaccines and substances injected into the body to start an immune response against cancer cells
- Non-specific immunotherapies that generally boost the immune system to enhance its anticancer activity

Although most patients who receive immunotherapies are not cured by these treatments, many patients are alive today or have survived significantly longer after receiving them.

However, to optimize your treatment, you still need to enlist immune system help.

It Starts in the Gut

The gastrointestinal tract is the body's largest immune organ and the main barrier between you and the 100 trillion microbes living inside you (your intestinal microbiome) plus any toxic substances you consume.

A diversity and balance of beneficial gut organisms helps maintain an anti-inflammatory environment; conversely, low microbial diversity or an overgrowth of pathogenic organisms can cause intestinal inflammation. And when your gut microbiome is compromised, chemotherapy and immunotherapy may not work as well.

Many things can kill off the beneficial microbes or foster unhealthy bacteria in the gut (dysbiosis), such as:

- Certain medications, including antibiotics, immunotherapies, chemotherapy, steroids, NSAIDs, and acid blockers
- Eating too many high-glycemic carbohydrates
- Not eating enough fiber or prebiotic foods (see below)
- Eating a lot of ultra-processed food
- Frequent eating; grazing
- Lack of dietary variety
- Food sensitivities or allergies
- High salt intake
- Fried foods
- Alcohol consumption
- Poor sleep
- Chronic stress
- Lack of physical activity
- Smoking
- Toxins, pesticides, and certain preservatives in food and water

To restore a healthy microbial balance in the gut, it's helpful to eat foods that contain beneficial bacteria (probiotics) as well as foods that nourish these (prebiotics).

Probiotics

Fermented foods and drinks that contain live bacteria include yogurt, kefir, and sour cream/crème fraiche made from animal or plant milks, raw fermented sauerkraut and pickles, drinks like kombucha and water kefir, and miso and tempeh.

Probiotic supplements can also supply beneficial bacteria. However, in view of the thousands of different probiotic supplements on the market, it can be hard to know which one is right for you.

Dr. Lawenda often recommends Sun Genomics' probiotic (sungenomics.com) to his patients. This company makes customized probiotic supplements based on an individual's stool sample. Every few months, the test is repeated and the supplement is modified as needed to address gut dysbiosis. While studies report the effectiveness of supplemental probiotics, it's very important to note that some data indicates potentially harmful effects. Check with your cancer care team before taking a probiotic supplement and ask whether you can safely eat foods containing live bacteria. If they advise against this, do what you can to consume prebiotic-rich foods.

Prebiotics

Prebiotics are certain types of fibers and starches found in foods that feed the gut's beneficial bacteria. Prebiotics meet three criteria:

1. Resistant to stomach acid, digestive enzymes, and gastrointestinal absorption
2. Fermented by intestinal bacteria
3. Selectively promote the growth of healthy intestinal bacteria

Prebiotic compounds are found in:

- Onions, leeks, garlic, chives
- All members of the cruciferous vegetable family (cabbage (all types), broccoli(ni), Brussels sprouts, kale (all types), radishes, arugula, etc.)
- Asparagus
- Avocado
- Banana, plantain (especially when less ripe)
- Bitter greens like dandelion greens, endive, and radicchio
- Eggplant
- Jerusalem artichokes (sunchokes)
- Jicama
- Honey
- Legumes (beans, lentils, chickpeas)
- Whole grains (e.g., oats, barley)
- Resistant starch from cooled and parboiled rice; cooked and cooled potatoes, cooked and cooled legumes (soaked or sprouted), tiger nuts
- Coconut meat and flour
- Foods rich in polyphenols such as chocolate/cocoa, coffee, fruits and vegetables (especially those with deep red and purple colors, such as berries, red cabbage, etc.)

It's not always easy to get enough prebiotic fiber from these foods, because some contain relatively small amounts. So, focus on getting enough fiber per day (25 g for women and 38 g per day for men), and consider taking a prebiotic fiber supplement like inulin. Based on research, 5 g of inulin a day boosts the growth of the good probiotic *Bifidobacteria* in your gut. (If you have gut symptoms like GERD, bloating, gas, diarrhea, or constipation, prebiotics can make these worse. If you want to take a prebiotic supplement, start with a small dose and increase gradually.)

Gut Problems

A growing number of people are afflicted with gut problems loosely diagnosed as irritable bowel syndrome. Countless factors can cause these symptoms; the two we see most often are food allergies or sensitivities and an overgrowth of bacteria or yeast in the small intestine (known as small intestine bacterial overgrowth, or SIBO).

If you suspect allergies or sensitivities, try an elimination and reintroduction diet to pinpoint troublesome foods. For best results, adhere strictly to elimination diet instructions; we recommend the protocol in the *Autoimmune Wellness Handbook* by Mickey Trescott and Angie Alt. A nutrition professional can guide you through the elimination and reintroduction phases to make sure you stay well nourished throughout.

If an elimination diet doesn't yield answers (or you don't have the time or energy for it), Dr. Lawenda recommends an IgG and IgA food intolerance test called the Cyrex 10 Multiple Food Immune Reactivity Screen that picks up on more subtle food sensitivities. You can get this test through a functional medicine trained provider, or through Dr. Lawenda's website: https://ioeprogram.com/lab-tests.

If you think you might have SIBO—characterized by bloating, gas, stomach pain, acid reflux, diarrhea, or constipation—ask your doctor to order a breath test to diagnose this. If you test positive, SIBO can be treated with the help of dietary changes (for instance a low-FODMAP or elemental diet) and antimicrobial drugs or herbs. (For more information, visit siboinfo.com.)

Immune nutrients

In addition to a healthy balance of gut microbes, the immune system also needs a wide variety of other nutrients in order to work properly:

- **High-quality protein,** such as wild-caught fish and seafood, eggs, and meat, ideally grass-fed or pastured.

Plant proteins like minimally processed soy foods, legumes, and plant-based protein powders can provide adequate protein too, but this requires a little more planning. (See protein section on p. 96) Low protein intake can result in depletion of immune cells, inability of the body to make antibodies, and other immune-related problems.

- **Anti-inflammatory omega-3 fats**, such as those found in oily fish, walnuts, flaxseed, and chia seeds. Omega-3s improve the function of white blood cells that engulf and digest cancer cells, among others, and are associated with tumor inhibition.
- **Vitamins A, E, K, C, B5, folic acid, B6, B1, B2, B12.** Eating a wide variety of vegetables and fruits is the best way to get these vitamins, as well as minerals, antioxidants, and enzymes.
- **Minerals.** Zinc is a potent immunity booster and its deficiency can suppress T-cell function. Iron is needed for phagocytic cell functioning (phagocytes are cells that engulf and consume foreign material, such as microorganisms, and debris, such as dead tissue cells.) Iron is also needed for adequate antibody response. Copper is involved in the development of immune cells such as T-cells and phagocytic cells. Selenium and manganese support healing from inflammation and may stimulate the immune system. Again, before you take a supplement, check with your doctor.
- **Mushrooms.** In addition to their antiviral, antibacterial, and anticancer properties, mushrooms stimulate various key immune-system components, such as T-cells and natural killer (NK) cells, both of which combat cancer cells. If you don't like mushrooms, consider taking a mushroom extract. Processing medicinal mushrooms through hot water or alcohol extraction yields significantly greater concentrations of their therapeutic compounds than eating the whole mushroom. A mushroom extract called PSK has

been found to improve survival when used alongside conventional treatments for gastric, esophageal, colorectal, breast, and lung cancers. Consider a supplement that contains a variety of different mushroom extracts, but talk to your doctor first.

Should You Eat a Neutropenic Diet?

One class of white blood cells, called neutrophils, attack and destroy pathogenic bacteria after they enter the body. Some cancer treatments and cancers that affect the bone marrow can cause white blood cell counts to drop sharply, a condition called neutropenia.

Neutropenia puts you at greater risk for infection and can interrupt cancer treatments, so it's crucial to keep your immune system as strong as possible. Even a minor infection can quickly become serious. Call your doctor right away if you have any signs of infection, such as fever, chills, aches, stiff neck, problems with urination or vaginal discharge, redness or swelling in any area, or vomiting.

Back in the 1960s, doctors thought that the best way to protect neutropenic patients was to reduce their exposure to all bacteria. Patients were washed, shaved, and disinfected, given large doses of antibiotics, placed in germ-free plastic tents, and fed only cooked food. Sadly, these measures did nothing to reduce mortality rates from infection.

Plastic tents are gone now, but many oncologists still recommend a neutropenic diet—even though it lacks credible scientific basis. Indeed, the largest neutropenic diet study to date, in which an all-cooked diet was compared to one that allowed raw fruits and vegetables, found no difference in infection and death rates. Today, neither the Food and Drug Administration, the Centers for Disease Control, nor the American Cancer Society support the neutropenic diet.

Alas, many doctors still use the "better safe than sorry" rule; in one survey, 57% of pediatricians said they use the neutropenic diet. But when you restrict fruit and vegetable intake, you're starving the gut microbes that are the backbone of a healthy immune system!

If your immune system or white blood count need a boost, follow our healthy dietary guidelines (pp. 86–172). Eat only the freshest fruits and vegetables and wash them before use, especially if you plan to eat them raw. If you want to play it extra-safe, briefly blanch vegetables or fruits before you eat or juice them. Or buy bags of high-quality frozen vegetables and fruits, which are often already blanched.

Over to You: Immune-Support Action Plan

- Take good care of your gut flora; eat probiotic and prebiotic foods daily (ideally at every meal)
- Eat a wide variety of plant foods
- Eat adequate amounts of protein (see protein section on p. 96 to find out how much you need)
- Manage stress; try to get adequate sleep and daily physical activity (even gentle)
- Eliminate alcohol; stop smoking
- If your blood counts are low, make sure your food is as fresh and clean as possible; cook or blanch it before eating

Support Apoptosis

Your body in its infinite wisdom destroys and eliminates cells that are abnormal, damaged, or no longer needed so that they can be replaced with new, healthy cells. Apoptosis is a natural process that helps maintain the correct balance between cell death and renewal.

Cancer cells mutate in ways that allow them to avoid apoptosis and continue growing and multiplying out of control. Radiation and chemotherapy trigger apoptosis—programmed death—in cancer cells, killing them off so they no longer affect the body. Unfortunately, these treatments kill off healthy cells, too.

Certain foods and herbs contain compounds that encourage cancer cell death without affecting the normal functioning of healthy cells, including:

- Cruciferous vegetables
- Yellow, red, orange, and dark-green vegetables
- Onions and garlic
- Strawberries, raspberries, pecans, and hazelnuts
- Apples (especially red ones)
- Legumes
- Green tea and white tea
- Unsweetened cocoa, dark chocolate
- Capsaicin, the compound that makes chili peppers spicy
- Turmeric and its active compound curcumin
- Ginger
- Clove extract

But don't stop at these; the more fresh, unprocessed foods you eat, the more you'll support your body's own anticancer mechanisms, including apoptosis.

Slow Angiogenesis

To grow, a tumor needs its own blood supply to deliver nutrients and oxygen. The growth of new blood vessels to nourish a tumor is called angiogenesis. Anything that impedes this process is called anti-angiogenic.

Under normal circumstances, angiogenesis is a vital and healthy process that heals wounds and restores blood flow to injured tissues. As soon as healthy, new vessel growth is complete, the body sends inhibitory signals to halt it.

When this balance is disturbed—as with cancer—abnormal blood vessel growth results. These new blood vessels are fragile and leaky, which allows cancer cells to escape, enter the bloodstream, and relocate to new locations where they can form secondary tumors (metastases).

The best time to use anti-angiogenic compounds—pharmaceutical or natural—is before cancer grows and metastasizes. That's not much comfort if your cancer has spread, but even advanced cancers can be slowed by including natural anti-angiogenic compounds in the diet. Anti-angiogenic factors may also prevent any remaining cancer cells from growing into new tumors and creating a cancer recurrence—so you should continue eating an "anticancer" diet indefinitely.

What makes a food particularly anti-angiogenic is eating it every day, several times a day, so that you ingest a dose of phytochemicals every few hours that will nip even the smallest microtumor in the bud—a process called chemoprevention.

Here are just some of the anti-angiogenic foods that you should try to consume every day:

- Green tea
- Berries (notably strawberries, blackberries, raspberries)
- Citrus fruit (notably oranges, grapefruit, lemons)
- Apples
- Pineapple
- Cherries
- Red grapes, red wine
- Brassica vegetables (notably bok choy, kale)
- Soy beans
- Maitake mushrooms
- Turmeric
- Nutmeg
- Artichokes
- Lavender (included in herbes de Provence)
- Pumpkin
- Sea cucumber
- Tuna
- Parsley
- Garlic
- Tomato
- Olive oil
- Grape seed oil
- Dark chocolate

If you eat three meals a day and include just one of these foods at each meal, that adds up to more than a thousand cancer-fighting food choices each year. (Find out more about anti-angiogenic foods and the body's other defense systems in the book *Eat to Beat Disease* by William Li, M.D., founder of the Angiogenesis Foundation (angio.org). His TED Talk is a must-watch: ted.com/talks/william_li_can_we_eat_to_starve_cancer?)

Numerous medicinal herbs also exhibit anti-angiogenic properties, including:

- Aloe vera extract
- Curcumin (in turmeric)
- European mistletoe (*Viscum album*)
- Chinese skullcap (*Scutellaria baicalensis*)
- Resveratrol
- Proanthocyanidin (grape seed extract)
- Milk thistle (silybum marianum)
- Ginkgo biloba
- Quercetin
- Mushroom extract poria cocos
- Panax ginseng
- Various herbal extracts used in traditional Chinese medicine

As with all herbal and nutritional supplements, do not take these without consulting your oncologist.

Over to you: Apoptosis and Angiogenesis Action Plan

- Broken-record alert: Eat a wide variety of plant foods—vegetables, fruits, herbs, spices, nuts, seeds, and legumes. Every day. At every meal. Indefinitely.

Consider Fasting

So far, we have talked a lot about eating. However, more and more integrative doctors recommend not eating for specific periods of time, also known as fasting—one of the world's most ancient healing traditions.

Research shows that fasting can help lower inflammation, oxidative stress, and insulin resistance and reverse type 2 diabetes and obesity, all well-known risk factors for cancer. Fasting also gives your intestines a break from the hard work of digestion, which helps to improve microbiome diversity and can calm bothersome gut symptoms.

Moreover, fasting can make cancer cells more responsive to chemotherapy while protecting the body's healthy cells. It can also help the immune system fight cancer that is already present.

Intermittent fasting (also called intermittent calorie restriction or time-restricted feeding) is an eating pattern where you voluntarily alternate between periods of eating and periods of not eating. The most popular methods include:

- **16/8 fasting:** This involves skipping breakfast and restricting your daily eating period to 8 hours, such as 11 am to 7 pm, and fasting for 16 hours overnight.
- **24-hour fast:** Also called "Eat–Stop–Eat," this involves fasting for 24 hours once or twice a week (for example, not eating from dinner one day until dinner the next day).
- **5:2 diet:** With this approach you consume only 500–600 calories on two days of the week but eat normally the other five days.

Cancer Protection

Studies of laboratory animals and humans who fast intermittently show clear improvements in a wide range of indicators:

- Reduced blood glucose and insulin levels, an associated increase in insulin sensitivity

- Reduced abdominal fat with maintenance of lean muscle mass
- Reduced levels of inflammation and oxidative stress
- Reduced blood pressure and resting heart rate, and increased heart rate variability
- Improved mood and cognitive function

Fasting is slowly gaining traction in the cancer community. For one, it may lower the risk of developing cancer in the first place, or risk of cancer recurrence in survivors. In one study, breast cancer survivors who didn't eat for at least 13 hours overnight—not such a stretch—had a 36% lower risk of recurrence and were 21% less likely to die of breast cancer.

In addition to creating an inhospitable environment for cancer cells, fasting can improve treatment response, protect healthy tissues against chemotherapy, and reduce treatment side effects, as illustrated in the chart below.

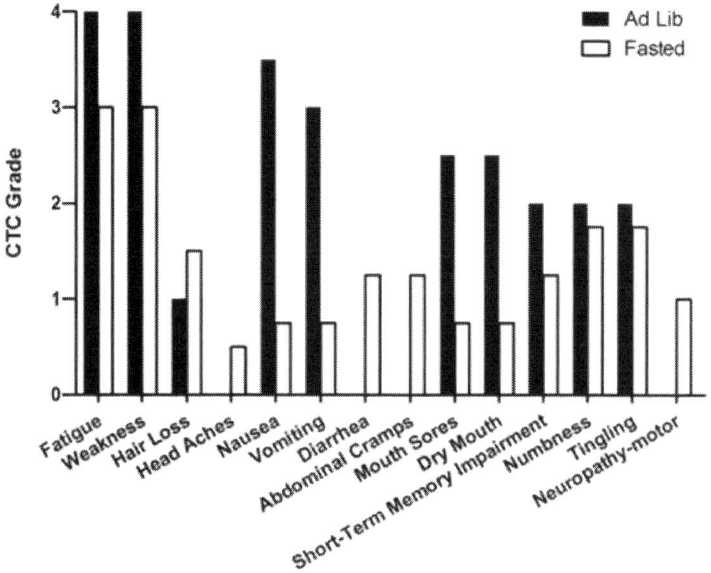

Figure 2: Fasting and cancer treatment in humans: A case series report by Valter Longo et al., Aging, 2009 Dec; 1(12): 988–1007.

Cautions

Concerns remain around fasting for people with cancer, notably regarding loss of weight and muscle mass. Considering that an estimated 80% of people undergoing cancer treatment are malnourished and experiencing muscle loss, skeptics point out that only a small number of patients may benefit from fasting. Some researchers also worry that calorie restriction or fasting may activate a process called autophagy that may promote cancer progression in certain circumstances.

Do not fast if you:

- Are underweight (BMI < 18.5) or actively losing weight
- Are pregnant or breastfeeding—you need extra nutrients for your child
- Are a growing child or teenager
- Have a history of disordered eating

You should fast only under medical supervision if you:

- Have diabetes mellitus, type 1 or type 2
- Take prescription medication
- Have gout or high uric acid
- Have any serious medical conditions, such as liver disease, kidney disease, or heart disease.

Before you embark on time-restricted eating, prepare for the following possible side effects:

- Hunger. This is usually less of an issue if you're eating a lower-carbohydrate, higher-fat diet.
- Constipation. Magnesium citrate supplements, hydration, and exercise may help.
- Headache, dizziness, mental fog, and fatigue. These are common and often due to low sodium, potassium, and magnesium levels, which get released through the urine during fasting. Add a pinch of salt or electrolytes to a glass of water a few times throughout the day, or drink bone broth or vegetable broth. (See also the section on electrolytes on p. 147.)

- Insomnia and anxiety. When we start to fast, adrenaline levels rise, which can cause jitters, anxiousness, and sleep disruption. Focus on your sleep hygiene (see p. 213).

If you're interested in adding fasting to your cancer treatment protocol, research your options carefully and ask your oncologist to help you weigh the potential pros (reduced treatment side effects and improved outcomes) and cons (weight loss, muscle wasting).

If you decide to give it a try, make sure you are monitored closely by a healthcare professional. A nutrition expert can help you ease into fasting and deal with any side effects you might experience. Apps like Zero (zerofasting.com) or Fastic (fastic.com) can help you track your progress.

Over to You: Fasting Action Plan

- Track how long you currently fast overnight and between meals. If your overnight fast is shorter than 12 hours, start by doing this: increase it by 5 minutes a day (by finishing dinner earlier or having breakfast later) until you reach 12 hours. Don't rush this process; your body and mind need time to adapt to changes in routine. (Read "Intermittent Fasting for Beginners," dietdoctor.com/intermittent-fasting.)
- Read *The Longevity Diet* by Valter Longo, PhD, particularly chapter 7, "Nutrition and Fasting-Mimicking Diets in Cancer Prevention and Treatment." (Dr. Longo has developed a 5-day fasting-mimicking diet product, Prolon; for more information, see prolonfmd.com.)
- Share these resources with your doctor and discuss whether fasting is appropriate for you.

Chapter 5

Move Your Body

Without a doubt, exercise is one of the most important things you can do to make your body less hospitable to cancer cells, thus reducing risk of cancer onset and recurrence.

Physical activity benefits everyone, but particularly people with cancer. We're not talking about Ironman triathlons, just good old-fashioned movement: walking, jogging, strength training, stretching, yoga, gardening, dancing, or even an energetic session with your vacuum cleaner.

Before starting any exercise program, get assessed by an exercise specialist to check your strength, balance, any weaknesses or limited range of motion, and other conditions that you need to factor in. Then work with a fitness trainer. You can find a Certified Cancer Exercise Trainer through the American College of Sports Medicine (certification2.acsm.org/profinder).

How Much Exercise

If you don't currently exercise, set a modest goal to start with and slowly work your way up. For instance, a good starting goal would be to walk for 15–20 minutes at a moderate pace. Once you're comfortable doing this, gradually increase the length and pace of your walks; walking briskly for 30–45 minutes a day is a great goal to strive for. For maximum cancer protection, longer and harder bouts of physical activity help. In one study, breast cancer survivors who briskly walked about one mile per day reduced their risk of dying from breast cancer by 24%; running for two-thirds of a mile each day reduced their risk by 40%; and running 2.3 miles per day cut their risk of recurrence by a whopping 95%.

Work up to the equivalent of at least 150 minutes per week of moderate-intensity aerobic physical activity (something that gets your heartbeat up, such as walking) or 75 minutes of high-intensity physical activity (where it's hard to talk without getting short of breath), using these guidelines:

- **Start slowly.** Jumping straight into a strenuous exercise routine can cause stress and injury. Work up to the degree of physical activity that makes you feel energized, but not exhausted. Aim for consistency.
- **Start simply.** Walk more often. Park your car further away from the store when you shop or run errands. Carefully walk a few steps on escalators; walk up a few flights of stairs before taking the elevator to your floor.
- **Find enjoyable activities.** Try to keep an open mind—there might be an activity you really like if you give it a chance. Consider karate, weight training, elliptical exercise machines, stair steppers, aerobics classes, Pilates, yoga, tai chi, qigong, squash, tennis, cardio training, or Miranda Esmonde-White's body conditioning exercises on Essentrics.com.

Muscle Mass Matters

Studies indicate that the greater your muscle mass, the lower your risks of dying from the most common causes of death in U.S. adults, including heart disease, diabetes, dementia, and cancer. Building and maintaining muscle tissue requires two key ingredients: dietary protein (see p. 96) and resistance exercise.

Get at least two days of muscle-strengthening activity per week—anything that makes your muscles work harder than usual, such as simple body-weight exercises (like squats, lunges, pushups, and planks) that you can do in your living room or kitchen (for instance, while waiting for the kettle to boil).

You can also work out with weights—either at the gym or at home—but do this safely, to avoid injury; it's best to begin weight training with the help of an experienced instructor who can show you how to safely perform exercises that are appropriate for you. Pilates, yoga, and Essentrics are also muscle-strengthening, though in more subtle ways.

And here's good news: You can work out only one day per week and get as much, if not more, muscle-building benefits as working out multiple days per week. Research shows that doing a single set of a resistance exercise once a week using heavier weights, with slow and controlled movements, over 90–120 seconds until muscles are totally fatigued builds muscle mass similarly to working out with multiple sets at lower weights, multiple days per week. (For more on this, check out the book *Body by Science* by John Little and Doug McGuff, M.D.)

Getting Started

Once you've decided to become more active, follow these guidelines to make sure you're doing the kind of exercise that's most suited to your needs and abilities:

- Ask your oncologist for a referral to a physical therapist who is experienced in working with cancer patients and survivors; the PT will assess your range of motion, pain, strength, sensation, and get a history of your medical conditions, surgeries, and other treatments
- Start your exercise program with a fitness trainer who is experienced in working with cancer patients and survivors; let your trainer and PT know that you want them to discuss your limitations so they can help you achieve your goals safely and effectively; check the American College of Sports Medicine (acsm.org) database to find a Certified Cancer Exercise Trainer
- You can work out at home or at a gym, using your body weight, resistance bands, weights, or machines

Activity Trackers

Most people overestimate how active they are. Exercise physiologists recommend at least 10,000 steps (about five miles) each day for good health. That translates to about 100 minutes—just over 1½ hours. In truth, Americans barely walk more than the "sedentary" rate of 5,000 steps per day.

To track your daily activity, buy a pedometer or other type of activity monitoring device. You don't need to buy the most expensive one with every bell and whistle; a simple $20 clip-on step counter can work as well as an Apple watch. Whatever you choose should be comfortable and easy to operate—ideally, just put it on and forget it.

These devices aren't perfect, but they are getting better all the time at accurately detecting different types of activity and movement. And if they help to motivate you to move more, then they're doing their job.

You Can Do This!

The most important exercise step is getting started. Remember these main points:

- Allow yourself adequate time to recover after cancer treatment; getting back to your pre-treatment fitness level will take time
- Avoid long periods of inactivity during the day, as this is linked to worse health outcomes, even if you exercise every day
- Any exercise is better than no exercise—the more you move, the better for your health
- Even if you don't have the energy to engage in formal exercise, walk as much as you can, stand up and stretch regularly throughout the day, throw in a squat or two while you're waiting for the kettle to boil, or sit on the floor when watching TV—anything to keep your body moving

Over to You: Exercise Action Plan

- Before starting any exercise program, get assessed by an exercise specialist, and then work with a fitness trainer.
- Buy a step-counter (pedometer) and track how many steps you currently take. Increase this number by a few steps every day. You'll be amazed by how quickly your step count will increase, and how much better you feel as it does!
- Support muscle strength; start with simple body-weight exercises and gradually work your way up.
- Move throughout the day; try to make it fun. Walk, run, skip, jump, duck, bend, lift, climb, dance, etc., whenever the opportunity arises. (Like playing with your (grand)kids, carrying laundry upstairs, carrying your groceries into the house, sitting and stretching on the floor while watching a movie, dancing to your favorite tunes, etc.)
- Get an exercise buddy to help you keep moving.
- Listen to music, a podcast, or an audiobook while exercising; this will make your workouts feel easier and more fun.
- Give yourself a big high-five when you've completed a workout. Research shows that celebrating even small wins motivates us to repeat new habits we're trying to adopt.

Chapter 6

Weighty Matters

Being underweight or overweight can adversely affect your health, especially when you have cancer. Unfortunately, cancer treatment often contributes to weight gain or loss, so in this chapter we suggest ways to address both.

Excess Body Fat Linked to Increased Cancer Risk

According to the CDC, excess body fat is associated with increased risk of at least 13 different types of cancer, estimating that these cancers accounted for about 40% of all cancers diagnosed in 2014.

Women are especially at risk: about 55% of cancers diagnosed in women (compared with 24% of those diagnosed in men) are related to excess body fat (cdc.gov/mmwr/volumes/66/wr/mm6639e1.htm).

Here's how the American Institute of Cancer Research (AICR) explains the link between excess adipose (fatty) tissue and cancer risk:

- Carrying too much body fat can produce proteins called cytokines, which trigger inflammation and/or chronic inflammation. Cancer happens when cellular growth becomes corrupted. A state of constant cellular growth with chronic inflammation creates more opportunities for such corruptions and cancer to occur.

- Having a large amount of adipose tissue can cause your body to produce too much estrogen, which can lead to the development of several cancers, including breast cancer and endometrial cancer.
- Fat cells produce a variety of proteins that cause high levels of insulin and other hormones, which in turn may spur cancer cell growth.
- Risk for cancer increases with excess visceral fat and significant excess body fat.

Even Modest Weight Loss May Cut Cancer Risk

If you think you may be carrying excess adipose tissue, we suggest you address this once you have finished treatment. That's because the more body fat you carry, the more likely you are to die of cancer—any cancer. Compared with death rates for men and women of healthy weight, cancer death rates are 52% higher for very obese men and 62% higher for very obese women (pubmed.ncbi.nlm.nih.gov/12711737).

Conversely, when people lose even a modest amount of body fat, their cancer risk may drop. One study found that women over 50 who lost 4.4–10 pounds over a period of 10 years had a 13% lower risk of breast cancer than women with stable weight. Women who lost 10 to 20 pounds had a 16% lower risk, and women who lost more than 20 pounds had a 26% lower risk (pubmed.ncbi.nlm.nih.gov/31845728).

Targeting Visceral Fat

Doctors usually assess their patients' weight in terms of body mass index, or BMI, which is based on a person's weight and height. However, BMI is a crude measure that says very little about our health. What exactly does the scale measure? Fat? Muscle? Retained water? BMI also doesn't take into account age, sex, or bone structure.

Even more critically, BMI doesn't identify *where* a person carries their fat—yet this differentiation is crucial. Some folks may have a high BMI because they're muscular or have fat stores in parts of the body where they are benign (for instance, the thighs or buttocks); even though they may be categorized as "overweight" by BMI standards, they may be metabolically healthy. Others might have a normal BMI, but carry inflammatory visceral fat (or belly fat) that puts them at elevated risk of insulin resistance and cancer (see p. 104 for more on the insulin–cancer link).

Visceral fat can be measured in various ways. CT scans and full-body MRIs are the most precise, but they are expensive and rarely available, so we like to use a simple, inexpensive method based on a person's waist circumference in proportion to their height. This is called the waist-to-height ratio (WHtR) and it can indicate whether you may be carrying excess visceral fat.

The WHtR is calculated by dividing your waist circumference by your height and multiplying the result by 100. The table below shows the WHtR ranges for men and women. For instance, a woman who is 65 inches tall and has a waist circumference of 31 inches has a WHtR of 47.7.

Table 3: Waist-to-Height (WHtR) Ranges for Women and Men

WHtR CLASSIFICATION	ADULT WOMEN	ADULT MEN
Extremely slim	≤ 34	≤ 34
Slim	35–41	35–42
Healthy	42–48	43–52
Mildly elevated	49–53	53–57
Elevated	54–57	58–62
Very elevated	≥ 58	≥ 63

Source: mdapp.co/waist-to-height-ratio-whtr-calculator-433

To calculate your WHtR, start by measuring your waist circumference:

- Do this first thing in the morning, before eating or drinking. Use a soft tape measure.

- Clear your abdomen of any clothing that might skew measurements. Stand in front of a mirror so you can check that the tape measure is straight and not twisted.
- Use your fingers to find the top of your hips and the base of your rib cage. Your waist is the soft, fleshy section between these two bony parts. It is typically the narrowest part of your torso and it is often located at or above your belly button.
- Exhale a normal breath.
- Wrap your tape measure around your waist so it is parallel to the floor. Don't pull too tightly or let the tape fall too loosely.
- Record your measurement.

Once you have measured your waist, calculate your WHtR by dividing your waist by height in inches and multiplying by 100, and check to see where it falls in the ranges shown in Table 3. If it exceeds the healthy range, consider taking action. But don't rush into a weight-loss diet; rather, work with your doctor to identify the factors that may have contributed to your waist gain.

There are dozens of reasons we store visceral fat, and they differ from one person to the next. For instance, your genes and ethnicity can predispose you to storing belly fat (Native Americans, Pima Indians, Hispanics, and those living in India and South Asia are more likely to have abdominal obesity).

Other factors include chronic stress, hormonal changes (e.g., menopause), lack of sleep and imbalanced gut bacteria. Sedentary lifestyles, diets high in refined and processed foods, excessive alcohol intake, and nutrient deficiencies can also contribute to visceral fat storage. Ironically, weight cycling (also known as yo-yo dieting) can drive insulin resistance and visceral adiposity, so more weight-loss dieting could be counterproductive.

The Holy Grail: Stick-with-ability

If you're reading this section, chances are you've tried a weight-loss diet (or several) over the years. Unfortunately, most weight-loss plans—especially those that promise rapid progress and entail calorie counting and intense exercise—don't yield sustainable results. They may work for a few weeks, but the honeymoon ends when calorie restriction causes muscle loss, fatigue, and depression, on top of constant, gnawing hunger, powerful cravings, and a rollercoaster of emotions. Sadly, dieters usually blame themselves when they fail, rather than their unsustainable diet plan.

To break out of the endless cycle of weight cycling and self-loathing, try to find ways to improve your metabolic health that you can stick with over the long term (i.e., for life!) There is no one method that works for everybody; in our experience, different approaches can be effective, provided you are able to stick with them.

Three Keys to Healthy Habits

So, what makes healthy dietary and lifestyle behaviors easy to stick with? Three factors: satisfaction, enjoyment, and patience.

Feeling fully sated by your meals can reduce the sense of deprivation many calorie-restricted dieters experience (and that often causes them to ditch their diets). Delicious meals that comprise high-quality protein, healthy fats, and fiber-rich foods like vegetables or legumes can deliver a deep and reassuring sense of satiety. Similarly, physical activity that engages your whole body and makes you feel good usually feels very satisfying.

Next, engage in healthy behaviors you enjoy—if you experience them as dreaded chores, they won't stick. Eat tasty meals that satisfy your body and your soul; move your body in ways that feel joyful and fun; undertake stress-relieving activities that feel uplifting and pleasant; and create calming rituals and an inviting space that make you look forward to bedtime.

Lastly, be patient, and don't make losing weight your primary objective. Rather, focus on integrating enjoyable, satisfying behaviors into your life as ends in themselves. Besides, when you regularly eat nutritious food, move your body in ways you enjoy, learn to manage your stress, and enjoy regular, restful sleep, you may find that your body composition changes and your lab results improve, even if you don't lose a lot of weight!

Target Hormones, Not Calories

When we counsel clients carrying excess visceral fat, we don't talk about calories; instead, we emphasize hormones—notably insulin, a hormone that regulates our fat stores, and cortisol, our body's main stress hormone.

We won't go into the hormonal complexities of fat metabolism here; there are many excellent books on this subject (we recommend a few in the appendix). However, here are some dietary and lifestyle measures that can optimize insulin levels:

- Eat a nutrient-dense diet (see p. 150)
- Eat high-quality protein at every meal (see p. 96)
- Eat nutritious fats at every meal (see p. 100)
- Eat vegetables, fruits, and legumes (nutritious and filling, thanks to their fiber content), and limit low-fiber carbs like sugar, pasta, white rice, etc. (see p. 109)
- Eat probiotic and prebiotic foods daily (see p. 180)
- Mindfully savor your meals
- Limit alcohol (see p. 237)
- Not eating for at least 12 hours overnight (see p. 189)
- Daily physical activity—even gentle (see p. 193)
- Adequate sleep and rest (see p. 213)
- Managing chronic stress (see p. 243)

Don't try to tackle all of these at once. Instead, start with a behavior that feels easy and pleasant, and work on it until it becomes automatic. This may take a few weeks. Then add another behavior, and so on. Adopting new habits—and letting go of old ones—takes patience, time, and practice; don't give up if you don't see immediate results. Focus less on your weight and more on adopting healthy behaviors you enjoy.

If this seems like an overwhelming undertaking, you might find it helpful to work with a nutrition professional, or join a support group (visit our websites to find out more). Working with others who are on a similar journey can make it easier to acquire new habits that support your health—and maintain them for the rest of your life.

Over to You: Adipose Action Plan

- Calculate your waist-to-height ratio (see p. 200). If it's elevated, ask your doctor whether now is the right time for you to make dietary and lifestyle changes.
- Identify factors that may have contributed to storing visceral fat. Some can be tackled fairly easily, others are harder to change. Start by working on the factors that are easiest to control; make sure this process is satisfying and enjoyable, and give it time.
- Be the tortoise, not the hare. Consider how long it took you to store the adipose tissue you're carrying and give your body time to adjust to your new behaviors. Don't pressure yourself, compare yourself to others, or beat yourself up when you slip or stall. Remain kind and compassionate with yourself throughout this journey.
- Consider joining a coaching and/or accountability group that follows the principles outlined here. Check our websites for more information.

Gaining Weight the Healthy Way

Some people are naturally thin, but healthy. In other cases, however, being underweight may increase your health risks. It can impair immune function, increase your risk of osteoporosis and fractures, and cause fertility problems. People who are underweight are also more likely to develop sarcopenia (age-related muscle wasting), and may be at greater risk of dementia.

Unfortunately, weight loss and being underweight are quite common in people with cancer, for various reasons: cancer treatments may reduce your appetite, change the way food tastes or smells, or make you too tired to prepare meals. Treatment-related side effects, such as problems with chewing and swallowing, nausea, or vomiting, can also put you off your food and this can lead to weight loss. (See pp. 25–80 for a detailed discussion of treatment side effects.)

Being underweight is defined as having a body mass index (BMI) below 18.5. (BMI is a more reliable measure when assessing low body weight than when assessing excess fat). This is estimated to be less than the body mass needed to sustain optimal health. You can calculate your BMI by using this calculator: calculator.net/bmi-calculator.html. Keep in mind that the BMI number is based on your weight and height; it does not differentiate between fatty tissue and lean mass (muscle, bones, etc.).

Several medical conditions can cause unintended weight loss, including thyroid problems, celiac disease, type 1 diabetes, infections, stress, impaired digestion and absorption, and eating disorders. If you are underweight, please ask your doctor to rule out a serious medical condition. If a medical problem is causing your weight loss, this needs to be addressed *before* you start a course of nutritional therapy for weight gain.

In some advanced cancer cases, people lose weight rapidly through muscle loss, a process called cachexia. This can be dangerous, because malnutrition weakens the immune system, raising the risk of life-threatening infections. Some 40% of cancer-related deaths are attributed to malnutrition caused by cachexia.

Cachexia stems from out-of-control inflammation, which reduces appetite and interferes with normal metabolism of nutrients. Individuals with cachexia need to pay close attention to eating enough protein and prioritize anti-inflammatory foods.

How to Gain Weight

Simply put: to gain weight, you'll have to eat more than you would need to simply maintain your weight. Cancer often increases your energy requirements, especially in people with advanced cancers.

As a rule of thumb, you should aim to eat an extra meal (roughly 300–500 calories) in addition to what you usually eat. It can be difficult to suddenly increase your calorie intake, especially when you're not hungry or are having digestive problems. Instead, gradually increase your portion sizes and meals to avoid indigestion and feeling overwhelmed. You can track your food intake on a food journaling app, such as Cronometer.

Eat Healthy Fats

If you are underweight, the best way to increase your energy intake is to incorporate healthy fats into your diet. That's because fat contains more than twice as many calories as do proteins or carbohydrates. While consuming protein will help you build muscle mass (when combined with some resistance exercise) and body weight, ratcheting up the amount of healthy fat calories in your diet can help you more quickly regain weight.

Here are some delicious, healthy ways you can increase your fat—and calorie—intake:

- Eat a tablespoon of unsweetened almond or coconut butter

- Add a hunk of cheese to your meal
- Hydrate with a glass of high-fat nut milk (such as hemp, hazelnut, macadamia, walnut, or coconut)
- Add a homemade protein shake to your breakfast or as an extra meal, using plant-based protein powders and high-fat nut milk
- Make cocoa or eggnog using high-fat nut milk
- Add heavy cream or high-fat nut milk to coffee or tea
- Drink a "bullet-proof" coffee blended with organic coconut oil, MCT oil, or powder, plus ghee or pure organic butter
- Add avocado to salads, soups, and stews, or spread it on crackers or toast
- Eat a bowl of berries covered with coconut cream (flavor this with a little stevia and vanilla extract, if you like)
- Use extra virgin olive oil for salad dressings; cook with olive oil at temperatures below 400°F; snack on olives
- Use high-quality avocado oil for higher-temperature cooking or salad dressings; use 100% avocado-oil mayonnaise; top salads, chilis or omelets with diced avocado
- Use coconut oil and ghee (clarified butter) for cooking, baking, and roasting
- Eat nuts (preferably raw and unsalted), nut butters, and nut oils
- Consume seeds (chia, flax, hemp, sunflower, pumpkin)—add these to smoothies, stir them into coconut porridge, or sprinkle them over salads and soups
- Use almond, walnut, hazelnut, macadamia, and MCT oils for salad dressings and in smoothies
- Savor Mediterranean dips and herb emulsions that contain olive oil, like pesto, salsa verde, hummus, roasted eggplant dip (baba ganoush) or tzatziki
- Enjoy dark chocolate, 75% cocoa content or higher
- Stir a few tablespoons of a healthy oil into hot drinks, grains, soups, and bean dishes
- Eat oily fish

- Add healthy oils or nut butters to smoothies, oatmeal or coconut porridge, mashed potatoes, salad dressings, and cooked or raw vegetables

And limit:

- Industrially processed fats, such as soybean, canola, corn, sunflower, and safflower oils
- Trans fats, found in margarines, hydrogenated oils, and processed and fried foods

Eat Protein for Muscle Mass and Strength

You need protein (see p. 96) to build muscle tissue and cells throughout the body—this is vitally important if cancer treatment causes lost weight and muscle mass (cachexia, see p. 205).

Healthy, high-quality protein foods include:

- Fish
- Meat
- Eggs
- Yogurt
- Beans
- Nuts and nut butters
- Protein powder

Eat Carbs for Energy

Minimally refined carbohydrates are a great source of minerals, vitamins, and fiber. They gently increase blood glucose (which provides energy) and insulin (which encourages fat storage and muscle synthesis).

Focus on nutritious carbs, such as:

- Vegetables
- Fruits
- Legumes (beans, chickpeas, lentils, etc.)
- Whole grains

Eat low-glycemic carbs at every meal, but don't overdo high-fiber vegetables, which can fill you up without providing many calories.

Avoid refined, processed carbs (sweets, pasta, white rice, soda, beer), which lack nutrients, can upset your blood sugar balance, and fuel inflammation.

Try to limit your total daily carbohydrates to 50–100 "net" carbs per day to reduce the swings in blood sugar and insulin that can fuel your cancer. (More on carbs on p. 104)

Optimize Digestion and Absorption

When you're trying to gain weight—especially if your appetite is low—having five or six small meals a day rather than three large meals can help. Chew your food thoroughly, and relax when you're eating. This helps your body break down and absorb more nutrients from the foods you eat.

If you can't chew or swallow solid food, drink your meals. Homemade smoothies, porridges, vegetable juices, and soups can provide easy-to-digest nutrients. Consult a nutrition professional for more ideas.

Chemotherapy may deplete digestive enzymes and healthy bacteria needed to digest food and absorb its nutrients. Digestive supplements can help; ask your doctor or a nutrition professional.

Mindful Meals

One way to stimulate your appetite and increase the nutritional health of your meals is to give yourself time and space to eat. That is, eat without distractions, focusing on your food—how it looks, tastes, and smells; take time to chew and swallow in small mouthfuls; and use mealtimes as a natural break in the day to refuel not only physically but also mentally and emotionally.

When you eat on the run, your body is in fight-or-flight mode and your digestive system doesn't work optimally, which can lead to malabsorption and nutrient deficiencies. When you relax and eat without distractions, you'll be in rest-and-digest mode, ready to absorb nutrients.

Eating as a Job

When working with people who are trying to gain weight, we often advise them to treat this process as they might a job, with schedules, plans, and targets.

For instance, rather than waiting to feel hungry before you eat, set reminders on your phone to help you remember to eat every few hours. Log everything you eat and drink on a food journaling app like Cronometer to make sure you're getting all the calories and nutrients you need. Appoint a "nutrition buddy"—a friend or family member—who can remind you to eat, help you shop for and prepare meals, and track your food journal entries.

It may also be helpful to make a weekly meal plan designed to get healthy fats, protein, carbs and probiotics into every meal. Planning doesn't mean cooking every meal from scratch; it simply means that you plan what and where you will eat. This can include restaurant meals, deliveries, ready-cooked meals or take-out—provided these contain protein, healthy fat, low-glycemic carbohydrate and, ideally, a nutrient-dense vegetable. A nutritionist or dietitian can help you design a meal plan that's suited to your specific needs and preferences.

Make Eating Easy

Choose easy-to-digest foods. Eat dishes with sauces and gravies, which are easier to swallow than dry foods. Shredded meat and gently cooked fish are easier to eat than meat that must be chewed thoroughly. Egg, tuna, and salmon salads are high-protein, high-calorie dishes that don't require much chewing.

Serve food cold or at room temperature to cut down on their odors, which can trigger nausea or loss of appetite.

Eat outdoors if you can, or make sure your dining room is well-ventilated, to cut down on food odors.

Work Your Muscles

Regular physical activity can support weight gain—in part because it may stimulate your appetite. You can maintain and build lean mass through weight training; begin lightly and increase weights slowly. As you start to recover strength, increase workout intensity gradually and add a little cardio training (walking, cycling, treadmill). None of this should be strenuous; ask a fitness trainer or physical therapist to design an exercise program that's appropriate for you.

Over to You: Weight Gain Action Plan

- Buy a cookbook or two, including Conner's *Zest for Life: The Mediterranean Anti-Cancer Diet* and the recipe books for cancer patients and survivors published by *Optimising Nutrition* (app.optimisingnutrition.com/cancer-recipe-books) that contain recipes for healthy, tasty meals.
- Assemble a nutrition support team to ensure you have constant access to nutritious foods. Enlist a friend to set up a rotation of people to shop and cook nutritious meals, ideally dishes that can be frozen so you can stock up, and steer them toward nourishing recipes.
- Talk to your care team as soon as any eating difficulties arise, either before or during treatment. Don't wait until you feel weak and have lost a lot of weight. Calculate how much you need to eat to gain weight (a nutrition professional can help).
- Write down a list of your five favorite fats (see our list on pp. 206–208)—make a point of eating one of these at every meal and add them to snacks.
- Eat high-quality protein at every meal.
- Eat minimally processed, nutrient-dense carbohydrate foods like vegetables, fruits and

legumes; blend and juice them if their fiber feels too filling.

- Eat frequent, small meals and chew your food thoroughly.
- Talk to a nutrition professional about ways to optimize your digestion and gut health.
- Start a gentle weight-training routine.

Chapter 7

Sleep and Circadian Health

Many people nowadays struggle with sleep—getting to sleep, staying asleep, or both—but people undergoing cancer treatment tend to be particularly affected by sleep problems. What's more, research is increasingly showing that poor quality or insufficient sleep raises our risk of developing conditions like cancer, diabetes, cardiovascular disease, and dementia.

In this chapter we take a closer look at the sleep–cancer connection and show you how to get the sleep your body needs to thrive.

Good Sleep for Better Health

Studies suggest that getting at least seven hours of nighttime sleep lowers cancer risk (as well as diabetes, heart disease, and obesity risks). Sleep deprivation, interrupted sleep, or exposure to light at night:

- Decreases the brain's production melatonin, a powerful hormone; decreased melatonin levels are linked to increased cancer risk
- May speed cancer growth, increase tumor aggressiveness, and dampen the immune system's ability to control or eradicate early cancers
- Produces more of the stress hormone cortisol, which stimulates tumor growth, metastasis (tumor cell

spread), angiogenesis (blood vessel growth), and reduces tumor cell death (see p. 185)
- Increases inflammation (see p. 174), which weakens the immune system, stimulates insulin resistance, boosts the production of tumor growth factors, increases free radicals, and impairs DNA repair

Pretty sobering, right? If, after reading this list, you want to take action to improve your sleep, here are some behaviors that can improve sleep.

Spend time outdoors every day. Daylight exposure—especially in the morning—stimulates the pineal gland in your brain, which triggers the production of melatonin. This hormone helps regulate your circadian rhythm and is a powerful antioxidant.

To function properly, the pineal gland needs daily exposure to daylight (without sunglasses). That doesn't mean staring into the sun, but simply being outdoors, for instance by walking while making phone calls, or sitting on a patio chair while meditating, reading, or enjoying your morning coffee or tea.

Spend at least one hour a day outdoors—although even 10 minutes is better than nothing—preferably before noon; wear a brimmed hat to shield your eyes if the sun is too bright.

Using a light box or light therapy glasses (such as the Ayo brand) can give you the same benefits as sunshine, without exposure to bright sunlight—useful if you live far from the equator. Studies show that you can improve your sleep quality by using light therapy for 30–90 minutes upon awakening each morning to help reset your circadian cortisol rhythm.

Blue Light. Exposure to blue wavelength light appears to be the primary culprit in disrupting melatonin production, especially during the latter part of the day. Blue wavelengths are especially prominent in computer screens, TV screens, and energy-efficient lighting (fluorescent and LED). Here's how you can reduce your blue-light exposure:

- Beginning two to three hours before bed, avoid looking at brightly lit screens (computer, smartphone, TV).
- If you work night shifts or use a lot of electronic devices, consider wearing blue-light-blocking glasses (our favorite brands are Swanwick, Felix Gray, and the more affordable Uvex). Installing a blue light filter, such as f.lux, on your devices, can help, too.
- Choose dim red light vs. white light for digital bedside clocks and night lights. Red light has the least power to shift circadian rhythm (see p. 213) and suppress melatonin. To reduce blue light exposure, use an alarm clock that has an amber, orange, or red light. This type of warmer light makes for a more restful sleep.

Rule out dental or breathing problems. If you wake up feeling unrefreshed or you're frequently tired during the day, your sleep may be getting disrupted by sleep apnea, bruxism (teeth grinding), or other imbalances. Discuss this with your doctor or dentist; they may prescribe a sleep study.

Use sleep-tracking technology. If you want data on how you're sleeping, the unobtrusive Oura ring device (ouraring.com) is worn on a finger to track sleep time and quality, heart rate, heart rate variability (a measurement of stress), and body temperature. If worn during the day, it also tracks activity.

Exercise. Exercising can help you sleep better. Get 20–40 minutes every day, ideally outdoors. Don't exercise after dark, except calming activities such as yoga or tai chi.

No caffeine after lunch. Stop caffeine intake at noon (or avoid altogether) if you're still not getting enough sleep. If you are used to having a lot of caffeinated drinks, stopping caffeine from one day to the next can be rough. We suggest you transition to a decaf lifestyle by initially combining decaffeinated with caffeinated coffee and tea (for instance, half a scoop of caffeinated coffee grounds and half a scoop of decaf grounds) and gradually increasing the decaf proportion until it makes up 100% of your drink. It's better to drink organic coffee, as non-organic is heavily sprayed with pesticides. When buying decaf coffee, choose one that's been decaffeinated through a non-solvent-based method (Swiss water or the more novel CO_2 process).

Free your mind. Before finishing work for the day, write down your most important meetings or appointments for the next day. This will reduce the amount of work-related fretting you do when you should be relaxing.

Cut out alcohol. Although alcohol makes most people sleepy initially, it often stimulates them a few hours later and disrupts sleep. It's also associated with a higher incidence of sleep-disrupting hot flashes.

Eat a well-balanced dinner. The brain needs all three macronutrients—protein, carbohydrate, and fat—to produce melatonin, so make sure your dinner contains a good amount of each. Eating a balanced meal can also help prevent blood sugar fluctuations during the night, a frequent cause of nighttime awakenings.

Wind down over dinner. No TV, radio, or computers; quiet, relaxing music is OK. Eat at a table, slowly and attentively. Say grace or go around the table inviting each diner to list one or two things they're thankful for, or take a moment of silence before you start eating. Avoid stressful topics of conversation. All of this not only aids digestion and absorption; calm, mindful eating can help lower overall stress levels and help you sleep better.

Take a short walk after dinner. Go alone to clear your thoughts, or with your partner to recap the day's events and reconnect. Post-meal walking lowers your blood glucose and helps you unwind. All it takes is 10–15 minutes.

Power down. Minimize or eliminate being in front of a screen 60 minutes before your desired sleeping time. Switch off your phone at least 60 minutes before sleep in a room that isn't the bedroom. Read a printed book or magazine rather than a laptop, phone, or electronic tablet.

Data dump. Thirty to 60 minutes before bedtime, quickly write everything that's currently on your mind onto an empty piece of paper and fold it up. This is not a to-do list; it's simply a place where you can park your thoughts or worries.

Journal your gratitude. Every evening, spend five or more minutes writing down three or more things that you're grateful for. Focusing on positive things—even if you have to force yourself to do it—allows you to take a step back from day-to-day worries and feel more optimistic about the future, thus reducing scope for nighttime rumination. (You can download a gratitude journaling template from Conner's website, modernmediterranean.com.)

Keep it dark. Make your bedroom as dark and quiet as possible. Use blackout blinds (especially during summer); cover any LED lights; replace ticking clocks with noiseless ones. Do not fall asleep to the sound of a switched-on TV or radio; their white noise may feel reassuring but will prevent you from attaining deep sleep.

Invest in comfortable bedding. Considering you spend about one-third of your life in bed, you owe it to yourself to use the highest-quality bedding you can afford. Sleep in breathable cotton sheets that can be washed at hot temperatures. Use comforters or blankets made from natural fibers and fillers that can be hot-washed, and seasonally appropriate bedding: lighter in the summer, warmer in winter. Buy a high-quality mattress. Get a pillow that supports your head and neck adequately.

Evict pets from your bed. Sleeping snuggled up to an adoring pet can feel wonderfully comforting, but if your four-legged friend encroaches on your space or wakes you up at night, you may need to set some boundaries. Train your pet to sleep on the floor, in a basket or crate next to your bed, or shut them out of your room at night.

Problem-solve with disruptive bedmates. If your partner is a noisy or restless sleeper, this can have a deleterious effect on your own sleep and health. A short-term solution can be to seek refuge in another quiet bedroom, if only occasionally. Ultimately, though, we recommend you and your partner investigate the causes of their problematic sleeping patterns and remedy these, where possible.

Don't just lie there. If you can't fall asleep after 20 minutes, get up and return to another space in the house to do a relaxing activity (under dim light), such as reading or listening to music. Lying in bed awake can create an unhealthy link between your sleeping environment and wakefulness. Instead, you want your bed to conjure only sleepy thoughts and feelings.

Wake up at the same time every day. Even if you have a hard time falling asleep and feel tired in the morning, try to get up at the same time, weekends included.

Avoid naps, if possible. Napping may cause sleep fragmentation and difficulty initiating sleep. If you need to nap, keep it short (around half an hour) and have them early, before 3 pm.

Keep your room cool. Sleep specialists recommend a room temperature of between 60–67°F. Your body temperature needs to drop to initiate good sleep. Temperatures that average in the 60s force your body to produce more melatonin, which facilitates falling and staying asleep. Consider a mattress pad, such as the Ooler Sleep System (chilitechnology.com/ooler), that circulates cool water (as low as 55°F) through a cooling unit.

Take a warm bath, shower, or sauna before bed. A warm bath of about 104–109°F for as few as 10 minutes can significantly improve overall sleep efficiency (more time spent sleeping rather than trying to fall asleep). Doing this one to two hours before bedtime can also speed up the time it takes to fall asleep by about 36%.

Practice slow, deep breathing. During nighttime waking periods, count your breaths. Count slowly to 10, then go back and start again. Or try the 4-7-8 Breath technique (see p. 74).

Rule out sleep apnea. If you or your sleep partner suspect that you might have sleep apnea (periods of not breathing in your sleep), talk with your primary care physician. This condition not only causes a disruption in sleep but can lead to other serious medical conditions that may undermine the health of your heart, brain, and metabolism.

Use alternatives. Other therapies that have been shown to improve sleep problems include acupuncture, aromatherapy, massage, yoga, and cannabis.

Learn Cognitive Behavioral Therapy for Insomnia (CBT-I). CBT-I is a technique that incorporates behavioral approaches to treat insomnia, either with or without medication. CBT-I helps you identify and replace thoughts and behaviors that cause or worsen sleep problems with habits that promote sound sleep. Unlike sleeping pills, CBT-I helps you overcome the underlying causes of your sleep problems. A CBT-I trained therapist will coach you through this program. One excellent CBT-I program is called Go! to Sleep, a clinically developed, six-week online course from the Cleveland Clinic that you can do in the comfort and privacy of your own bedroom (clevelandclinicwellness.com/gotosleep).

Mindfully meditate. Mindfulness meditation involves focusing on your breathing and then bringing your mind's attention to the present without drifting into concerns about the past or future. It helps you break the train of your everyday thoughts to evoke the relaxation response, using whatever technique feels right to you.

Guided sleep meditation can help you let go of worrying thoughts and relax your body before bed. Like other forms of meditation, this practice involves moving your focus away from your mind to sensations in your body. Regular practice of guided sleep meditation has been shown to improve sleep. If you have trouble meditating by yourself, you may find a meditation app helpful; many of these have special meditations for people struggling with sleep. Our favorites are Calm, Headspace, 10 Percent Happier, and Waking Up.

Get help. If you're plagued by persistent emotional problems or anxieties that keep you up at night, consider working with a psychologist or coach who specializes in sleep problems.

Over to You: Better Sleep Action Plan

- Determine why you are having trouble sleeping. Could it be your medications? Chronic stress? Looking at screens late at night? Caffeine, alcohol, and/or sugar consumed late in the day? Physical pain? Emotional distress? Discuss with your doctor and tackle as appropriate. (More on emotional distress on p. 239.)
- Try Cognitive Behavioral Therapy for Insomnia, either with a CBT-I therapist or through a self-guided program, like the Cleveland Clinic's.
- Get out into daylight (without sunglasses) every morning, as soon as possible after waking.
- Exercise daily, ideally outdoors.
- Eat balanced meals, especially at dinner, and ensure adequate protein intake.
- Switch off screens at least 90 minutes before bedtime. Use blue-light-blocking glasses if you're looking at screens in the evening. Keep the lighting in your home dim at night.
- Meditate.

Timing is Everything: Circadian Health

For optimum health, it may not be enough to sleep seven hours, eat well, and exercise. It's *when* you do all of these things that can have a powerful effect on health.

Humans have an internal timing system called the circadian clock. It's responsible for programming every aspect of physiology, including breathing, heartbeat, digestion, immune system function, detoxification, making new cells and hormones, and regulating blood pressure, temperature, blood sugar balance, and insulin production.

Because the body can't perform all these jobs at the same time, the circadian clock sets a specific, well-timed daily schedule for these activities. Disrupting the body clock—especially over long periods of time—is associated with increased cancer risk, especially colorectal, prostate, and breast cancer, and many other health conditions.

Unfortunately, modern living can make it difficult to maintain a healthy circadian rhythm. The most common circadian disruptors include:

- Irregular sleep schedule
- Bright light at night (lamps, computers, phones, tablets, night lights)
- Insufficient time spent outdoors
- Erratic eating patterns (eating over periods of more than 12 hours a day; snacking throughout the day)
- Caffeine, alcohol, and tobacco
- Not exercising, or exercising at suboptimal times
- Chronic stress

Sleep for Circadian Health

Sleep *quality* is as important as quantity. Here's how to achieve it (more about this in the previous section):

- Develop a sleep routine and don't diverge from it on weekends; go to bed at about 10 pm and wake up seven to eight hours later, ideally without an alarm

- Reduce bright light exposure in the evening
- Keep your bedroom dimly lit; try blue-light-free light bulbs and use blue-light blocking glasses
- When you wake up, quickly expose yourself to bright light; go outdoors as soon as possible to help reset your body clock

Eat for Circadian Health

It turns out that the adage "Breakfast like a king, lunch like a prince, dinner like a pauper" may be true. Dozens of studies show that blood sugar control is best in the morning and worst in the evening. The body also burns more calories and digests food more efficiently in the morning. Therefore:

- Eat a hearty breakfast that includes healthy protein, fats, and low-glycemic, high-fiber carbohydrates; these help you feel full and reduce the desire to snack.
- Avoid caffeinated drinks after noon, and avoid chocolate and cocoa at night
- Consume no calories, caffeine, or alcohol two to three hours before bed (water and herbal tea are OK); this helps the body do all its nocturnal work: detoxification, tissue repair, and growth, fat-burning, and more—it also helps you sleep better
- Fast for at least 12 hours overnight

None of this is etched in stone, so adapt these guidelines to your schedule. For instance, if the only way you can practice time-restricted eating is by breaking your fast at 11 a.m. or noon—a very popular practice among intermittent fasting practitioners—then don't force yourself to eat earlier. Experiment to find out what works best for you.

Exercise for Circadian Health

Physical activity of any kind triggers the production of certain molecules in muscles that activate the "muscle clock." This strengthens your circadian clock to help you sleep better.

Morning outdoor exercise—for instance, a simple half-hour walk or run—is great for stimulating your body clock, lowering inflammation, and burning fat. If you must exercise indoors, try to do it near a window.

Muscle tone rises in the afternoon, so this is a good time for weight-lifting and high-intensity exercise. Afternoon exercise also reduces appetite.

Exercising after dinner, such as a walk, can lower blood glucose and improve digestion. However, high-intensity exercise in the evening can increase your temperature, cortisol, and heart rate, and make it harder to fall asleep. If you exercise late, take a lukewarm shower to cool your body down.

Chronomedicine

Amazingly, timing can even influence the effects of surgery, radiation, or chemotherapy. Researchers in the emerging field of chronotherapy, also known as chronomedicine, are working to discover when to schedule treatments so that they provide the most benefit and do the least harm.

Since many drugs target receptors, enzymes, or proteins involved in cell-signaling pathways that are governed by the circadian clock, medications and treatments should ideally be delivered accordingly. Most of today's best-selling drugs work better when taken at specific times of day.

The largest cancer chronotherapy trial so far compared chronotherapy with conventional chemotherapy in 564 people with metastatic colorectal cancer. Survival times were similar in both groups, but when results were broken down by sex, the risk of an earlier death dropped by 25% for men, but increased by 38% for women. The researchers inferred that men best tolerate one type of cancer drug between four and seven hours earlier in the day than women do. Still, only 1% of ongoing clinical cancer trials incorporate time-of-day considerations, according to a 2016 survey.

For more information on circadian health:

- Read *The Circadian Code* by Satchin Panda, PhD, and take the circadian quiz. If you answer "yes" to any questions, optimizing your circadian system will benefit your health.
- Download the app My Circadian Clock (mycircadianclock.org) to track your circadian rhythm and find out which areas to tweak.
- To measure your light exposures and make adjustments, download smartphone apps myLuxRecorder (Apple) or Lux Light Meter (Android).

Melatonin and Cancer Treatment

We mentioned melatonin earlier—it's the hormone our body makes to help us fall asleep. In addition to this role, melatonin:

- Acts as an antioxidant
- Stimulates immune function
- Reduces inflammation
- Prompts cancer cell suicide (apoptosis)
- Protects nerve and immune cells
- Blocks growth of new blood vessels in tumors (angiogenesis)
- Decreases estrogen receptors and estrogen production in women and men

A review of human clinical trials using melatonin as a supplement in cancer patients found that those taking melatonin had significant improvements compared with those not taking it:

- 40% had a greater chance of being alive one year after diagnosis (both for patients undergoing and not undergoing chemotherapy)
- 233% (all patients) and 93% (patients taking chemotherapy) had a greater chance of having no tumor identified after treatment
- 90% (all patients) and 253% (patients taking chemotherapy) had a greater chance of tumor regression

- 51% (all patients) and 15% (patients taking chemotherapy) had a greater chance of no tumor growth or new metastases after treatment

Reassuringly (albeit based on limited data), melatonin appears to be safe during chemotherapy and radiation therapy without reducing treatment efficacy. Typical melatonin doses, taken 20 minutes to three hours before sleep, are:

- Low dose: 0.3 mg per day (used to help regulate sleep and to combat jet lag)
- High dose: 20 mg per day (used in cancer management in small studies)

Some practitioners recommend starting at the low dose and increasing to 20 mg over one to four weeks to minimize side effects, such as vivid dreams and drowsiness. As with any supplement, always discuss taking it with your oncology team first.

Chapter 8

Clean Up Your Environment

Cancer develops when changes in a cell's DNA cause the cell to grow out of control. Sometimes, these changes—or mutations—are caused by chemicals and other toxic substances in the environment, known as carcinogens because of their cancer-causing potential.

Toxic chemicals don't always cause cancer, however. Your risk depends on several factors—including how long and how often you're exposed, your genes, diet and lifestyle, overall health, age, and gender.

When it comes to environmental carcinogens, it may seem like avoiding exposure is as impossible as avoiding the air you breathe. In reality, though, you have more control than you think. Let's take a closer look at the exposures you can influence.

Overhaul Your Kitchen

Creating an environment in your body that's hostile to cancer involves minimizing exposure to any potential toxins. Start with where you eat.

Safe Pots and Pans

When equipping your kitchen, minimize the use of items that are made from or coated with man-made chemicals, such as:

- Plastic containers, especially when microwaving
- Nonstick pans, especially if overheated or scratched
- Teflon and some of its chemical components, such as PFOA
- Food cans or cartons lined with plastic or silicon

Also, avoid aluminum and copper pots and pans, which can leach aluminum (associated with nervous system disruption) and copper (thought to cause a copper–zinc imbalance) into food, especially acidic foods such as tomatoes. However, this is not a concern with stainless-steel pans that have an inner core of aluminum or copper to help conduct heat. Since the aluminum or copper is sandwiched between layers of steel and doesn't come into contact with the food, this type of stainless-steel cookware is fine to use.

Wherever possible, favor natural or inert materials: wood, earthenware, glass, stone, china, bamboo, stainless steel, and cast iron.

- **Stainless steel and enamel** are excellent cookware materials: safe, flavor-neutral, hard-wearing, and easy to clean. High-grade stainless-steel skillets are not prone to sticking and are easy to clean. You can use steel wool and metal implements in them. Stainless-steel pressure cookers, including the wildly popular Instant Pot, cook foods at a fraction of the time needed to prepare them in conventional pots and preserve more of the foods' vitamins and minerals.
- **Cast-iron or carbon steel** pans contain no synthetic materials, are extremely durable, and conduct heat evenly. To keep foods from sticking, cook at slightly lower temperatures. Once these pans are well-seasoned, food rarely sticks. To clean, soak briefly in water, and wash with a sponge or soft brush. Dry cast iron immediately to prevent rust.
- **Glass** (such as Pyrex) works well for oven-baked dishes and storage containers. They are also microwave-safe.

Ditch Plastic

Certain chemicals interact with the estrogen receptors on our cells and may play a role in the development of several endocrine disorders, including hormone-dependent tumors such as breast and prostate cancer. These chemicals include bisphenol-A (BPA), which is used to make plastic containers and the linings that coat the insides of food and drink cans, and phthalates, which are widely used in baby toys, food processing equipment, and medical devices.

Even at weak concentrations, BPA can block the effects of several chemotherapy agents on breast cancer cells. Low doses of BPA have also been found to promote the proliferation of thyroid cancer cells and testicular germ cell cancer in humans. Unfortunately, alternative materials developed by chemists, including bisphenol-S, which replaces BPA in many food cans, may be just as hazardous as BPA. Even the most minute concentrations (less than one part per trillion) of BPS can disrupt a cell's normal functioning.

The vast majority of plastics used in modern food processing—can linings, plastic wrap, sandwich bags, disposable water bottles, food storage containers, convenience-food packaging, water filters, and much more—contain chemicals that can leach into foods and may have adverse health effects. In one investigation, a research team found that 92% of all BPA-free kitchen plastics tested leached compounds into food they came into contact with, even when they were not being stressed (exposed to heat or light). Under stress, some 98% of plastics gave off these compounds.

Until more is known about safe levels of these chemicals, try to minimize your exposure to plastics:

- Instead of buying food that's tightly packaged in plastic, buy it loose and store it in glass or stainless-steel containers or wrapped in wax paper
- Use glass or stainless-steel containers for leftovers or fresh foods stored in the fridge and freezer
- Where possible, buy conserved foods in glass jars rather than cans

- Babies should drink from glass bottles; toddlers can use stainless-steel sippy cups; minimize canned formula or foods
- Drink filtered water from stainless-steel or glass bottles instead of plastic ones
- Boil water in stainless-steel or enamel stove-top kettles, or even a casserole with a lid
- Avoid drinks in cans (like soda), which are lined with plastic resins
- Buy a blender and food processor with glass jugs, especially if you use them to process hot foods
- Make coffee by pouring boiling water over paper filters in stainless-steel or ceramic filter holders; minimize coffee made in plastic coffee makers or from single-use plastic capsules
- Use ceramic, glass, or metal bowls to prepare food; for cooking, use stainless-steel, carbon-steel, or cast-iron pots and pans, and wooden, bamboo, or stainless-steel implements. Eat food on china, glass, ceramic, or earthenware plates. Use glass pitchers and glasses.

Drink Clean Water

Tap or bottled? Many consumers purchasing bottled water think they're buying a high-quality product. In reality, countless companies are simply filtering municipal water and bottling it—and the quality of this water is often far from desirable.

In a 2018 study, 93% of the 11 bottled waters tested contained microplastics—tiny pieces of plastic debris less than five millimeters in size. Bottled water can also contain residues of polyethylene terephthalate (PET), a chemical suspected of being able to alter our hormonal systems. Moreover, phthalates in plastic bottles can seep into the water, especially when exposed to high temperatures or stored for an extended period of time. Lastly, laboratory tests conducted in 2008 found that 10 popular brands of bottled water contained 38 chemical pollutants ranging from fertilizer residue to industrial solvents.

Unlike bottled-water companies, municipal tap-water suppliers must publish their water quality tests. Contact your local water supplier for their annual tap-water quality report. You can look up your city's report in the Environmental Working Group's National Tap Water Atlas (ewg.org/tap-water). If you use a private well, have it tested by a specialist laboratory.

For added protection, the EWG recommends filtering tap water. Carbon filters (pitcher or tap-mounted) are affordable and reduce many common water contaminants like lead and by-products of the disinfection process used to treat municipal tap water. The more expensive reverse-osmosis filters can remove some contaminants that carbon filters can't, like arsenic and perchlorate. Our favorite brand of water filters, Berkey, has been shown to remove more than 200 contaminants as well as bacteria and viruses (Berkeyfilters.com).

When using water filters, it is important to change the filters as often as their manufacturers advise; old filters can harbor bacteria and let contaminants through.

Are Microwaves Safe?

Many people believe that microwave ovens cause cancer—not helped by the fact that many of us use expressions like "nuking" or "zapping" to describe microwave cooking.

First of all: nothing obliges you to use a microwave oven—our ancestors managed fine without them. However, if you'd like to use one but are concerned about its safety, there is no scientific evidence showing that microwaves produce harmful radiation or cause damage to nutrients. If you follow some simple guidelines, microwaving is a safe and healthy cooking technique.

Microwave cooking involves waves of energy that cause water molecules in food to vibrate, producing heat that cooks the food. Because microwave cooking is faster than other cooking methods, vitamins that usually break down when heated, like vitamin C, are less affected than by other cooking techniques.

Microwave ovens are equipped with metal shields that prevent the radiation from leaving the oven, thus reducing risk. Microwave emissions are generally below the federally mandated level at a distance of two inches; leakage above that level is extremely rare. If you still feel nervous, simply step away from the microwave while in operation. If it doesn't close properly, replace it.

Some people worry that microwaving denatures nutrients in food. However, very minimal molecular changes happen with microwaving, due to the low energy waves given off. The only chemical or physical change that happens to food when it is microwaved is that its temperature increases.

Don't use plastic in microwaves; the ever-evolving science makes it uncertain whether plastics—even so-called "microwave-safe" ones—are completely safe. Instead, use nonreactive materials: glass, china, and ceramic. Instead of plastic wrap, cover microwaved food with a sheet of parchment paper, plain white paper towels, a glass lid, or an upturned plate.

Over to You: Clean Kitchen Action Plan

- Critically review your kitchen utensils and storage containers, and keep only those that are made from inert materials (glass, stainless steel, china, ceramics, wood, bamboo, etc.); phase out those made from plastic and replace them with non-reactive substitutes
- Research the quality of your local tap water
- Invest in a water filter; maintain it carefully
- Phase out plastic water bottles and replace them with stainless steel or glass water bottles
- Toss out scratched nonstick pans

Replace Toxic Cleaning Products

Laundry soap, toilet cleaners, scrubbing powders... the cleaners you use every day could be adding to your toxic load.

Search the EWG's Guide to Healthy Cleaning (ewg.org/cleaners) to find "greener" options for all your household needs, decode technical terms on labels, and more. You can buy toxin-free household cleaners at health food stores and online co-ops like Thrive Market (thrivemarket.com).

If you like DIY projects or live on a tight budget, you can even make your own home-cleaning products.

Over to You: Home-Cleaning Action Plan

- Pull out all of your home cleaning products and look them up on the EWG's website (EWG.org/cleaners); throw out any that score poorly
- Research less-toxic replacements on the same site
- Research and make your own home- and laundry cleaning products. The internet is a goldmine of information—we also like the book *The Naturally Clean Home: 150 Super-Easy Herbal Formulas for Green Cleaning*, by Karyn Siegel-Maier

Detoxify Personal Care

Cancer loves inflammation, free radicals, and tumor growth hormones—all of which may increase when you use certain personal care products (makeup, shampoo, soap, lotion, perfume, toothpaste, deodorant, sunscreen, etc.) on your body.

Research indicates that although many of the chemicals commonly used are "safe" when tested individually, when combined they can cause cancer. Here are just some of the commonly found cancer-promoting compounds in many of our personal care products:

- BHA/BHT
- PEGs
- Petrochemicals
- Parabens
- Phthalates
- Formaldehyde releasing agents
- Siloxanes
- Sulfates
- Fragrance/perfume

Go through all your personal care products—cosmetics, shampoos, soaps, lotions, perfumes, toothpaste, deodorants, sunscreens—and exchange the unsafe ones with more healthful alternatives. Here are three fantastic tools to help you decide which to keep and which to ditch:

- **ThinkDirty** (thinkdirtyapp.com). Use this app to learn about the safety of thousands of personal care products. You can even scan the barcodes on product labels to access the product database.
- **Skin Deep** (ewg.org/skindeep), an online cosmetics safety database created by the Environmental Working Group. This searchable database rates more than 78,000 personal care products.
- **EWG Guide to Sunscreens** (ewg.org/sunscreen), a comprehensive database.

Over to You: Body Care Action Plan

- Go through all your body care products and look them up on one of the apps listed above; get rid of any that score poorly.
- Search the same apps for nontoxic replacements
- Research and make your own body care products—we like Stephanie Tourles' 2007 book *Organic Body Care Recipes: 175 Homemade Herbal Formulas for Glowing Skin & a Vibrant Self*

Spa Safety

Going to a spa can be a comforting experience for anyone undergoing or recovering from cancer treatment.

Before booking your appointment, though, let your care team know that you'd like to go to a spa or see a spa therapist. Ask about any recommendations or limitations. Check that your spa therapist is trained in Oncology Esthetics (oti-oncologytraining.com) or Oncology Massage Therapy (s4om.org).

Use these common-sense guidelines for your next spa visit:

- Just because a product looks or says "organic" or "natural" doesn't mean it's necessarily safe for you. Discuss skin care products with a specialist or esthetician who has experience working with cancer patients.
- Avoid massage that uses heat or friction in the areas undergoing cancer treatment, unless approved by your oncologist.
- Hygiene is critically important. Make sure your spa therapist explains how they disinfect all equipment, surfaces, tools, and water baths. If sanitation standards are not to your liking, find another spa. Your skin is very vulnerable to infections during cancer treatment, so you need to be vigilant.

Over to You: Safe Spa Action Plan

- If you like spa treatments, ask your care team whether they're safe for you
- Ask them to recommend a trustworthy spa that employs certified oncology massage therapists and estheticians
- Only go to a spa if you're feeling well
- Enjoy getting pampered; you deserve it!

Green Your Garden

If you're a gardener, and especially if you grow your own vegetables (two activities we enthusiastically encourage!), think twice about the chemicals you use to make your garden grow.

Remember Monsanto's Agent Orange, used during the Vietnam War to kill off jungle plants? Despite many protests, complaints, and lawsuits, it wasn't until years later that Agent Orange was identified as responsible for causing numerous cancers and other disabling diseases.

For years, chemical companies disputed a link between pesticides and cancer. But a 2013 study published in *CA: A Cancer Journal for Clinicians* definitively concluded that pesticide exposure through food, water, skin, and air increases cancer risk, particularly:

- Breast cancer
- Prostate cancer
- Leukemia
- Lymphoma
- Multiple myeloma

Numerous plant- and weed-killing chemicals in common herbicides have also been clearly established as carcinogens. These chemicals can cause cancer by:

- Increasing the production of free radicals
- Acting as endocrine disruptors, which block or mimic the actions of hormones
- Increasing the activity of cancer-promoting genes or decreasing the activity of cancer-suppressing genes

Disturbingly, many of the culprit carcinogenic pesticides and herbicides are fat soluble, which means they can stick around in the body for years.

What can you do?

- Become more aware of known carcinogens and potential carcinogens
- Identify the ways in which you are exposed to them
- Minimize your exposure

By all means, garden—it's great for your health, offering physical activity, daylight, fresh air, and connection with the earth and the seasons. Also, don't stop eating fruits and vegetables simply to limit exposure to pesticides. In fact, eating lots of fruit and vegetables actually reduces your risk of cancer, and if you grow them yourself, they'll likely be fresher than any produce you can buy. Just make sure you're not inadvertently exposing yourself or your food to toxic chemicals.

Over to You: Safe Gardening Action Plan

- Find out whether any of your garden chemicals contain banned substances (azchemistry.com/list-of-banned-garden-chemicals); if they do, dispose of them carefully
- Research chemical-free/organic gardening methods
- Manual labor and tools such as rakes and garden hoes can offer an alternative to chemicals when it comes to maintaining your lawn or garden (and provide a great workout!)

Quit Tobacco

Smoking, including the inhalation of second-hand smoke, is a leading cause of cancer and death from cancer. This applies to *all* tobacco products—cigarettes, vapes, cigars, pipes, hookahs, bidis, kreteks, chew, and snuff.

The risks from smoking are even worse if you have the following cancers:

- With bladder cancer, your risk of dying is 295% greater if you smoke
- With lung cancer, your risk of dying is 236% greater if you smoke
- With colorectal cancer, your risk of dying is 231% greater if you smoke

Smoking during radiation therapy and chemotherapy also decreases the effectiveness of those treatments. Smoking delays wound healing after surgery and increases surgical complications. And smoking makes cancer pain more severe.

Obviously, it's best never to take up smoking, but even if you do, it's *never too late* to stop—all the more so if you've been diagnosed with cancer. According to one study, quitting smoking even after a cancer diagnosis helps you live significantly longer than those who don't quit.

Over to You: Smoking Cessation Action Plan

- Go to the NCI's Smokefree.gov website and use the Step-by-Step Quit Guide
- Call the tollfree NCI Smoking Quitline at 1–877–44U–QUIT (1–877–448–7848) for individualized counseling, printed information, and referrals to other sources
- Check out the NCI fact sheet *Where to Get Help When You Decide to Quit Smoking* (cancer.gov/about-cancer/causes-prevention/risk/tobacco/help-quitting-fact-sheet)

Alcohol Alert

While compounds in red wine, such as resveratrol, anthocyanidins, and procyanidins, are powerful antioxidants, the ethanol in alcoholic drinks contributes to several common cancers, including those of the breast, mouth and throat, and esophagus; some research also links it to liver and bowel cancer. The risk of some alcohol-related cancers is even greater in smokers.

While a moderate intake of alcohol, notably red wine, may reduce heart disease risk, the same protective benefits do not extend to cancer. Indeed, according to research, the more a person drinks regularly over time, the higher their risk of developing cancer.

Alcohol increases cancer risk by:

- Breaking down the ethanol in alcohol to acetaldehyde, a toxic chemical and probable carcinogen
- Generating free radicals that can damage cells' genetic material
- Impairing the body's ability to break down and absorb cancer-protective nutrients
- Increasing blood levels of estrogen, a hormone linked to breast cancer risk

If you want to enjoy the healthy plant compounds in red wine (e.g., resveratrol, anthocyanidins, and procyanidins) without the carcinogenic ethanol, these can be obtained from foods such as cocoa, apples (especially Red Delicious, Granny Smith, and Reinette), cranberries, grapes, raspberries, pomegranates, persimmons (also known as kaki or Sharon fruit), nuts (especially walnuts, but also almonds and hazelnuts eaten with their skins), mulberries, cinnamon, and tea.

Over to You: Safe Alcohol Action Plan

- Decrease your alcohol intake with a view to eliminating it altogether
- If you are dependent on alcohol, join an alcohol treatment program; to find out about different treatment options, visit the National Institutes of Health's Alcohol Treatment Navigator website: alcoholtreatment.niaaa.nih.gov

Chapter 9

Healing Mind and Spirit

If you have been diagnosed with cancer, it is natural to experience a bucketful of emotions.

You may experience shock, fear, anxiety, panic, or a combination of all of these. As the news sinks in, and you go through the rigors of treatment, questions may arise, such as "How did this happen?" and "Why me?"

At some point, most people diagnosed with cancer—even those who have completed treatment—will experience at least mild symptoms of depression; many will experience a deeper sense of sadness and symptoms of moderate to severe depression. Almost all cancer patients and survivors experience mild, moderate, or severe stress, anxiety, and fear in response to diagnosis and treatment.

This is borne out by research. A 2014 study published in the *Journal of Clinical Oncology* found that one in three of the 2,100 patients in cancer care centers in Germany experienced anxiety, depression, or other mood disorders—a higher prevalence than in the general population. And a 2013 study published in the *Lancet*, evaluating 43 studies involving 51,381 cancer patients, found that long-term cancer survivors are more likely to experience anxiety than their spouses or the general population.

These emotions may last for only a few days or weeks, or they may become a longer-term conditioned response that affects everyday life. If they become more deeply embedded in our psyches and are experienced over a longer time period (e.g., months or years, not just weeks), it is important to recognize these changes and get help when needed.

Address Depression

Over the past two weeks, how often have you been bothered by any of the following problems? (0 = Not at all, 1 = Several days, 2 = More than half the days, 3 = Nearly every day)

- Little interest or pleasure in doing things
- Feeling down, depressed, or hopeless

If you score three or more points on both questions, tell your cancer care team or primary care physician.

Being depressed while undergoing or recovering from cancer can worsen outcomes:

- Minor or major depression increases risk of premature death in cancer patients by up to 39%; patients displaying even few depressive symptoms might be at 25% increased risk of mortality.
- Recurrent exposure to emotional distress could diminish natural killer cell function, implicated in tumor cell control
- In hormone-related cancers, depression could negatively affect multiple cancer defense processes
- People with distress symptoms are more likely to smoke, be sedentary, eat a less than healthy diet, and become obese—thus increasing their cancer risk
- Depression can disrupt sleep, the gut microbiome, and genes that normally suppress tumor formation, thus creating an environment in which cancer can thrive

How Depression Feels

People undergoing cancer treatment often describe depression as a weight. Others describe depression as being drained of all physical energy, even enough to perform simple day-to-day tasks. Some describe feelings of helplessness or hopelessness.

Often, individuals describe depression as a "black hole" that blocks their ability to feel any sense of pleasure in the activities and events that once gave them joy. Smell, taste, touch, hearing, and sight may become blunted. Depression may also feel like numbness—an inability to feel at all.

When someone receives a diagnosis or cancer, they may experience the loss of their personal life story as they believed it to be. Many cancer survivors describe the process as becoming "story-less." In other words, their interpretation of who they are and what they believed their life would or should be like has been dramatically altered.

Before diagnosis, they felt in control of their lives. Now, their days may be filled with doctor's appointments and treatments, with financial challenges, and with physical limitations during or after treatment ends.

Although your story will be changed, there is every potential for the plot to become richer than it was before. The transformation that occurs in people facing life-threatening events is often described as "benefit finding"—seeing meaning or purpose in what is happening. This can help you move forward after cancer in ways that make life even more meaningful than it was before your diagnosis.

Depression After Treatment

Post-traumatic stress disorder (PTSD) and its related depression most often occur six to eight weeks after cancer treatment has ended. Why?

People who have completed cancer treatment will tell you that while they were in treatment, their medical providers and others, including themselves, were busy saving their life and closely watching their medical status. There was comfort in knowing that everything was being done to produce the best medical outcome.

Once treatments end, a different stage of recovery begins. There's more time to think about the big questions: "Why did this happen? Was it something I did? What should I do now?"

There's also the fear of recurrence. When you're no longer being medically watched on a daily or weekly basis, even the most diffuse and innocuous symptoms—an ache here, a twinge there, a feeling of fullness, an unfamiliar swelling—can be taken as a sign that the cancer is back.

If cancer treatment lasts for years, as with metastatic disease, the risk of depression is even greater because treatment fatigue often sets in. Even though stage 4 cancer can be treated and managed long term within a high-quality life, the journey can erode emotional and physical resources.

It's critically important to develop and maintain strategies for relieving long-term emotional distress, including depression. If you feel depressed or anxious, see a psychologist who specializes in cognitive behavioral therapy, or CBT. CBT can significantly reduce or eliminate anxiety, depression, stress, and PTSD caused by diagnosis of and treatment for cancer.

Over to You: Depression Action Plan

- If you think you might be depressed, take the depression quiz (above). If your score is 3 or more, talk with your doctor and ask them to refer you to a mental health professional.
- Try to stay connected with others. For instance, talk about your feelings with someone you trust. Have lunch or coffee with a friend. Help someone else by volunteering. Ask a loved one to check in with you regularly. Go to the movies, a concert, or a museum with someone. Call or email an old friend. Go for a walk with a friend. Schedule a weekly dinner date. Take a class or join a club.
- Do things that make you feel good. For instance, spend some time in nature. Read an uplifting novel or poetry. Watch a lighthearted movie or TV show. Take a long bath. Play with a pet. Talk to friends

or family face to face (including by video call). Listen to music that lifts your spirits. If it's got a good beat, dance to it.

- Research shows that many of the lifestyle habits described in this book, such as eating a Mediterranean diet, having healthy gut bacteria, undertaking daily physical activity, being outdoors, getting adequate sleep, and having a support network of caring people, can ease depression. Try to integrate these into your life over time. If you don't know where to start, work with a coach.

Manage Stress

You probably understand intuitively the link between stress and the immune system. After all, how many times have you come down with a cold shortly after an episode of high stress?

Now, imagine what your body goes through when exposed to stress over years. Humans evolved to deal with temporary and passing stress, such as the stress of finding food, water, and shelter. These are quite different from the constant stresses of modern life, from financial pressures and deadlines to relationship difficulties and nonstop news.

Substantial evidence suggests that exposure to chronic stress increases rates of cancer development and growth. New research indicates that stress can cause permanent changes to genes, including those that perform key controls in the cancer process.

Once a tumor has developed, stress hormones can make things worse by:

- Increasing tumor growth rates, tumor cell invasiveness, metastatic activity, and tumor blood vessel growth
- Suppressing natural killer (NK) cell activity
- Reducing effects of chemotherapy on tumor cell apoptosis (cell death)

Are you stressed?

Stress manifests in many different ways, including:

- Constantly feeling tired and run down
- Regular bouts of digestive or intestinal discomfort (bloating, acid reflux, diarrhea, constipation, etc.)
- Regular head, back, or neck aches
- Sore jaw, teeth grinding
- Inexplicable skin breakouts or flare-ups of eczema, psoriasis, dermatitis
- Hair loss
- Trouble concentrating
- Trouble sleeping
- Regularly feeling anxious, angry, depressed, helpless, out of control, impatient, forgetful, hostile
- Being easily irritated
- Comfort eating, drinking more than seven alcoholic beverages a week, drinking a lot of coffee, smoking heavily
- Rushing around without getting anything done, feeling overworked, procrastinating

Go through this list and score the stress symptoms that you experience regularly. If you score more than three, you are probably experiencing elevated stress.

Managing Stress

Whether you have cancer or not, stress is inevitable and out of our control. However, what we *can* control is how we respond to the stressors life throws at us.

Evidence linking chronic stress, immunity, and cancer is mounting. An important study in 2008 found that stress was associated with higher cancer incidence in initially healthy populations (6–21% increased risk) and higher risk of dying of cancer (29–133% increased risk). Conversely, one study that followed 227 breast cancer patients over 11 years found that women who received stress-reduction support had a 59% reduced risk of dying from breast cancer.

A cancer diagnosis itself causes harmful stress: In one study, investigators found that for 6,500 adults who survived childhood cancers, 9% (nearly 600 individuals) reported signs and symptoms consistent with PTSD. Further complicating this picture, stress often leads to high-risk behaviors, such as smoking and excessive alcohol use, poor diet, lack of exercise, and obesity, that increase cancer probability. Stress also disrupts sleep and circadian rhythms, which is linked to an increased incidence of certain cancers.

The takeaway: Dedicate at least 30 minutes every day to reducing stress. Strategies abound and include breathing techniques such as 4-7-8 breathing (p. 74), counseling, support groups, exercise, acupuncture, guided imagery, supplements, botanicals such as CBD (p. 81), and many more. Here, we look more closely at yoga, massage, meditation, biofeedback, and sauna.

Yoga

A 2019 review found that for cancer patients and survivors, yoga:

- Reduces salivary cortisol (stress hormone) levels, improves emotional well-being, and reduces fatigue after cancer treatment
- Improves post-treatment disturbances in sleep and cognition
- Reduces cancer-related fatigue and improves vigor
- Improves biomarkers of stress, inflammation, and immune function
- May improve symptoms of anxiety, depression, pain, cancer-specific effects such as lymphedema, and psychological outcomes

Yoga also can alleviate many cancer treatment side effects, both during and after cancer treatment, by improving circulation and respiratory capacity and by helping you cultivate self-awareness, presence, and compassion.

Not all yoga instructors are prepared to provide modifications without some advance warning, so contact the studio or instructor before your first visit to discuss needs or limitations. If possible, find an instructor who specializes in yoga for cancer patients. For one-on-one instruction, ideal for students dealing with post-surgical or chronic health, pain, or mobility issues, consult with a Certified Yoga Therapist (find one on iayt.org or y4c.com).

Here is a list of precautions compiled by yoga teacher and cancer coach Ellen Fein:

- Ask your medical team if there are any yoga postures that you shouldn't practice immediately after surgery.
- Because your immune status makes you more vulnerable to illness and infection, the room, mats, and props must be clean. Bring your own clean sheet or blanket from home, so you don't have direct contact with the floor. If you're in a therapeutic yoga class, any students with cold, flu, or infection symptoms should not come.
- Cancer treatment can cause low blood platelet counts, which can lead to bruising and bleeding. Avoid props such as resistance bands and yoga straps that apply direct pressure to the skin.
- If you have a port or central line that delivers drugs directly into a vein, your doctor may advise you to limit certain physical movements, especially those where the head is lower than the heart (for example, the downward-facing dog pose). Other doctors impose no restrictions, so be sure you understand your doctor's instructions. Always err on the side of caution.
- Tumors or radiation can make bones vulnerable to fractures, especially in the spine, pelvis, or ribs. Avoid any yoga postures that stress the bones, including anything that uses leverage or torque (seated twist, bound triangle, bound side angle, and most hand-to-big-

toe variations). When in doubt, keep your yoga practice as gentle as possible.

- Lymphedema, a common cancer treatment side effect (see p. 52), causes fluid accumulation, typically in the arms or legs. Avoid long holds of poses that extend the affected limb overhead. Move in and out of such a pose briefly. Avoid putting direct weight on the affected limb.
- If you feel any pain, numbness, shortness of breath, or dizziness during yoga practice, ease off immediately and come out of the pose to a resting state. (There is no such thing as "work through the pain" in yoga.) Alert the instructor or ask for help if the symptoms persist.

Massage

Massage has become one of the most popular complementary treatments used by cancer patients, thanks to its physical and emotional benefits. While not curative, massage can:

- Reduce the side effects caused by surgery, chemotherapy, and radiation therapy
- Improve mood and ease depression
- Reduce stress and anxiety
- Provide pain relief
- Improve appetite and control nausea
- Alleviate fatigue and improve sleep
- Promote blood and lymph flow
- Break up scar tissue
- Promote faster wound healing
- Improve range of motion and mobility

An oncology massage can be quite different from a regular massage. For one, you'll be asked to complete a detailed intake form to ensure maximum safety. Standard oncology massage intake questions cover:

- Your cancer treatment history
- Tumor site or metastasis
- Compromised blood cell counts
- Lymph node involvement

- Blood clots or blood clot risk
- Medications (short and long term)
- Vital organ involvement
- Fragile or unstable tissue
- Medical devices
- Fatigue, neuropathy, or pain
- Changes in sensation
- Late effects of treatment

In addition to providing this information, keep these things in mind:

- If you're undergoing chemotherapy and radiation, do not have a deep-tissue or strong pressure massage, which can cause bruising
- If you're undergoing radiation, ask your massage therapist to avoid touching any sensitive skin or any temporary markings in the corners of the radiation treatment field; if you don't have skin irritation in the treatment area, massage may be done very lightly through a soft towel or cloth
- If your lymph nodes have been removed, tell your massage therapist to use a very gentle touch on your affected arm and the area around the underarm
- If you have arm lymphedema, the massage therapist should avoid the affected arm and underarm areas; traditional massage therapy can worsen lymphedema, so find a specialist in lymphedema massage, called manual lymphatic drainage

Meditation

Effective, safe, and free, meditation can significantly reduce the production of stress hormones, help reverse the physiological effects of stress that make the body more conducive to cancer, and improve your quality of life. It is scientifically proven to be effective and requires little more than a comfortable, quiet space.

For you, the word "meditation" may conjure images of bearded yogis seated cross-legged on mountain tops. But today's approaches to meditation are decidedly more modern, with user-friendly apps available on smartphone stores and YouTube. Our favorite meditation apps are:

- 10 Percent Happier (tenpercent.com)
- Calm (calm.com)
- Headspace (headspace.com)
- Insight Timer (free) (insighttimer.com)

Biofeedback

To get visual feedback on your body's reaction to stress or relaxation, you can use a heart rate variability (HRV) tracking device while you perform breathing exercises (see p. 74 for 4-7-8 breathing) or meditation.

HRV measures beat-to-beat irregularity. The greater your heart rate variability, the more your parasympathetic nervous system (relaxation system) is dominant. That's a good thing; higher HRV is associated with better cancer outcomes and quality of life.

With an HRV biofeedback device such as Inner Balance (heartmath.com/innerbalance), the ear clip monitor sends real time HRV readings to a free downloadable app on your smartphone. As you relax, the app shows you how you're doing. It can be highly motivating to watch your stress melt away before your very eyes.

Sauna

The Finnish tradition of sauna, long used for pleasure and relaxation, may offer several health benefits. For instance, HRV has been shown to increase after sauna bathing, which translates to lower stress. A number of small studies indicate other health-promoting effects, including:

- Decreased "bad" LDL cholesterol and increased "good" HDL cholesterol

- Reduced inflammation
- Improved heart and immune system function
- Reduced blood pressure
- Reduced anxiety and depression
- Reduced risk of Alzheimer's disease

While traditional saunas heat up the surrounding air to about 185°F, infrared saunas only reach about 140°F. Infrared rays penetrate more deeply into the body, which means you start sweating at a lower temperature than in a traditional sauna (and you can enjoy a longer session without overheating).

Infrared sauna:

- Beginners: 5–10 minutes at a time, three to four times a week
- Maximum: 30–60 minutes at a time, five to seven times a week

Dry (Finnish) sauna:

- Beginners: 5–10 minutes at a time, three to four times a week
- Maximum: 15–20 minutes at a time, five to seven times a week

Moderate sauna use appears to be safe for most people. However, if you have cardiovascular disease, speak to your doctor first. When sauna bathing, make sure you remain well hydrated, as sweating can cause dehydration. People with certain conditions, such as kidney disease, may be at a higher risk of dehydration. The increased temperatures can also lead to dizziness and nausea in some people.

Installing a sauna at home can be costly; before you make this investment, try sauna bathing at a gym or spa to see if you like it.

Over to You: Stress Management Action Plan

- Accept that there are parts of your life you cannot control; try to let go
- Focus your thinking on the positive; keeping a gratitude journal can help
- Practice meditation, breathing techniques, yoga, or other relaxing activities
- Try to get 7–8 hours of sleep between 10 pm and 6 am
- Undertake physical activity every day to boost endorphins and relieve mental and physical tension
- Connect with people you care about and who make you happy
- Avoid negative self-talk; have compassion and patience for yourself, even when you may not be performing up to your usual standards—often, "good enough" is just fine
- Eat calm sit-down meals on a regular food cycle (breakfast, lunch, dinner—ideally with people whose company you enjoy) and minimize caffeine, especially after lunch
- Consider each request for your time or attention, and sometimes say no
- Make time for yourself; put "me time" on your calendar
- Seek support from a certified mental health professional to process any traumatic experiences or relational difficulties in your life, past or present

Music Therapy

Many people with stressful medical conditions use music as a therapeutic intervention: It's cheap, easily accessible, nontoxic, and can make you feel better almost instantly.

Studies show that listening to music helps lower anxiety, fatigue, and depression during cancer treatment. As recently as April 2016, a study found that singing in a choir for just one hour boosts levels of immune proteins in people affected by cancer, reduces stress, and improves mood. Many integrative cancer centers encourage their patients to use music to help them cope with pain, mood swings, depression, anxiety, nausea, and vomiting. In fact, some centers offer music therapy.

Music therapy isn't about learning to sing or play an instrument. In a music therapy session, you may simply listen or move to music, sing, play with simple instruments, write or discuss song lyrics, take a gong bath, or use guided imagery alongside music.

Music therapy can also help alleviate suffering as people approach the end of life. Some music therapists, musicians, and singers perform at the bedside of ill and dying people to help ease their transition and to offer solace to loved ones.

While most types of music are pleasant, not all of it is therapeutic. For instance, celebrities performing at hospitals, a piano player in the clinic lobby, nurses playing background music for patients, or a choir singing on a hospital's pediatric floor are not considered therapeutic. As the American Music Therapy Association defines it, music therapists:

- Assess emotional and physical well-being, social functioning, communication, and cognitive skills through musical responses
- Design music sessions based on client needs using improvisation, listening, songwriting, lyric discussion, imagery, performance, and learning through music
- Participate in interdisciplinary treatment planning, evaluation, and follow-up

To find a credentialed music therapist near you, consult the American Music Therapy Association at musictherapy.org.

Over to You: Music Action Plan

- Create playlists on your favorite music streaming platform that contain your favorite composers, genres, and instruments. Perhaps create different lists for different moods.
- Sing, sing, sing! For instance, by joining a choir, singing along to your favorite songs, or using a karaoke app like karafun.com.
- Dust off your old guitar or teach yourself a simple instrument like the ukulele, the recorder, percussion instruments, or a set of bongos
- Make music with others, not (necessarily) to perform, but just to have fun; you can find bandmates through local music schools, musician finder sites like musofinder.com or bandfinder.com, online forums like CraigsList.com or reddit.com/r/FindABand, or via social media
- If you like classical music, listen to Swiss National Radio's 24-hour commercial-free classical music station at radio.net/s/swissclassic

Writing Therapy

For some, processing feelings through the written word gradually eases emotional trauma. Writing therapeutically can be done individually or in a group, in person with a therapist, or remotely through mail or the internet.

Initial findings suggest that writing down your thoughts and feelings every day can:

- Reduce stress
- Boost the immune system

- Improve the mental and physical health of cancer patients
- Release the "feel good" hormone dopamine
- Help you overcome negativity and clear your mind—especially when you throw away the paper afterward

You don't have to take a course in creative writing to derive the benefits of journaling. Just buy a large notebook or create a document on your computer and get started. Be sure to keep it in a safe place; privacy is crucial for writing without self-censoring.

Blogs have become a popular way for people to process their cancer journey. Indeed, some cancer centers have started hosting patient-authored blogs on their websites as clinicians begin to recognize the therapeutic value.

Blogging offers the added benefit of reaching readers in similar situations and creating supportive communities. It can also provide a nifty way to stay connected with friends and family without having to call or email. CaringBridge.org, for example, is a nonprofit platform that allows you to set up a personal website, giving you one centralized, private place to share health updates and request help.

Meanwhile, try to journal daily for about 20 minutes, either on paper or on your computer. Don't worry about spelling and punctuation. Write quickly, stream-of-consciousness style.

An article in *Coping Magazine* suggests a number of ways to journal:

- Art journaling: draw or scrapbook what you are feeling
- Dream journaling: write down the first two or three words that come into your mind when you wake up; these words can help you to recall your dreams
- Gratitude journaling: write down the things you are grateful for; this enables you to focus your attention on positive aspects of your life

- Humor journaling: find the humor in a situation and write about it; comedic outlets can help improve your mood
- Line-a-day journaling: limit yourself to just one sentence per day
- Stream-of-consciousness journaling: write down whatever comes to your mind as you are thinking it; it's OK if it comes out nonsensical

If you don't know where to start, pick a theme for the day, week, or month (for example, "peace of mind," "transition," or "resilience"). Or use journaling prompts—the internet is full of them—such as:

- What am I grateful for today?
- When am I at my happiest?
- Three things I value about myself are....
- I feel most energized when....
- A thank-you letter to someone you love

If journaling doesn't feel helpful, or brings up painful memories, don't push it; try something else.

Over to You: Writing Action Plan

- Join a journaling program to get you started; we like psychotherapist Michelle Chalfant's free 30-day journaling challenge (theadultchair.com/30days-old/)
- Create a blog on CaringBridge.org or MyLifeLine.org, where you can share your cancer journey with friends and family
- Gratitude journaling: write down the things you are grateful for—this enables you to focus your attention on positive aspects of your life, and can be particularly helpful for anyone experiencing anxiety or depression

- If you don't have much time or energy to spare, try "line-a-day" journaling: limit yourself to just one sentence per day
- If you find writing hard, try art journaling (copingmag.com/art-meditation-for-the-cancer-journey/)

Laugh

For someone living with cancer it may seem hard to find humor when facing such a serious medical condition. Yet, laughter is natural medicine.

Indeed, a growing body of research indicates that laughter has therapeutic value. Laughter therapy, also called humor therapy, aims to use the natural physiological process of laughter to help relieve physical or emotional stress or discomfort.

Over the years, researchers have found that laughter episodes help to:

- Reduce pain and stress-related hormones
- Boost the immune system
- Decrease anxiety, depression, tension, and rage
- Ease insomnia
- Improve lung function

When used in conjunction with conventional cancer treatments, laughter therapy:

- Has major positive effects on quality of life, resilience, immunity, anxiety, depression, and stress
- Boosts the activity of the body's natural killer (NK) cells, which keep tumor cells in check

Cancer Treatment Centers of America offers humor therapy sessions, also known as Laughter Clubs or humor groups, to help cancer patients and their families use laughter as a tool for healing. During these exercises, it's hard for people not to join in, because laughter is so contagious.

Over to You: Laughter Action Plan

- Watch a funny movie or TV show
- Watch stand-up comedy at a club, on TV, or on the internet
- Read the jokes and cartoons in newspapers or magazines; clip any you particularly like and post them where you'll see them daily
- Seek out people who make you laugh (and avoid those who drag you down)
- Share a good joke or a funny story
- Check out your bookstore's humor section
- Host game night with friends
- Play with a pet or goof around with your kids or grandkids
- Go to a laughter yoga class (laughteryoga.org)
- Look up Bianca Spears' laughter yoga videos on YouTube—she'll have you giggling in no time
- Do something silly, like singing to yourself in a public place, laughing out loud at the movies or in a restaurant, or wearing something completely out of character
- Make time for fun, mindless activities, such as bowling, miniature golf, or karaoke

Cultivate Connection

When confronted with a cancer diagnosis, most people turn to the people closest to them: a spouse, sibling, parent or adult child, close friends and neighbors, or fellow members of social or religious communities. Reactions can vary, including minimizing ("Oh, I'm sure you'll be fine,") or catastrophizing ("Oh no, how terrible!"). But most people simply feel at a loss as to what to do or say.

This is where you can and should get proactive. Rather than leaving family and friends guessing, clearly ask for the sort of support you need. This is a research-backed strategy: studies show, for example, that women with large, high-quality social networks and support have better chances of surviving breast cancer than those with smaller networks.

Tell people what you need from them. Ask them to read this chapter. Direct them to *Holy Shit, You've Got Cancer (A Quick-Start Guide)*, a free ebook by psychiatrist and cancer survivor Elana Miller (available at zenpsychiatry.com; click on "Resources," then on "Newsletter and Free Resources" and sign up to download the guide) that includes a detailed list of do's and don'ts on supporting someone who has cancer.

What to Say to Friends and Family

Here are some clear requests that you can communicate to your loved ones:

- Just be there for me. I don't expect you to fix my problem, offer advice, or make me feel better. I just want you to be fully present with me and listen when I need to talk.
- Make plans with me, be it a visit to the movies in two weeks' time or a camping trip next summer. This will give me something to look forward to during some of the darker hours of my cancer journey. Keep plans flexible in case something comes up or one of us needs to cancel or reschedule.
- Laugh with me and allow me to be sad. Be humorous and fun when appropriate and needed. A light conversation or a funny story can make my day. But don't ignore uncomfortable topics or feelings.
- Check in. Text or call me every two to three days just to let me know you're thinking of me. Don't be offended if I don't pick up; I may not be in the mood to talk, but that doesn't mean I won't be delighted to hear from you.

- I am not my cancer. I still have interests, wishes, hopes, and dreams. Please treat me the same as before, and let's not always talk about cancer—I need a break now and then!
- Read my blog or group emails. Dip in once or twice a week to stay current with my updates so that I don't have to repeat experiences or information multiple times.
- When you don't know what to say, it's better to say, "I don't know what to say," than to stop calling or visiting out of fear. Here are some other things you can say (or write in a card) to show your support: "I'm so sorry this has happened to you." "If you ever feel like talking, I'm here to listen." "How can I help?" "I care about you." "I'm thinking about you."
- Here's what *not* to say or write, please: "I know just how you feel." "Here's what you should do." "You absolutely *must* try this supplement / diet / clinic / treatment." "Don't worry, you'll be just fine." "How long do you have?"

Some people have trouble asking for help, which leaves even the most well-meaning supporter at a loss. When someone asks you "Is there anything I can do?" it's fine to be assertive and ask them to do specific tasks for you. You could even post a list to your Caring Bridge page or send them out in a group email entitled "Ways You Can Assist Me."

Here are some suggestions:

- Shop for groceries (I'll send you my shopping list and reimburse you)
- Pick up prescriptions
- Pick up books from the library
- Help with chores around the house
- Cook a meal and drop it off at my house; I'll send you a recipe that suits my current dietary requirements (please make extra so I can freeze half for another meal)
- Babysit my child(ren), take them to and from school and activities, or arrange for play dates

- Organize a phone chain and/or support team to check on me regularly
- Drive me to an appointment or a support group meeting; offer to take notes during an appointment or provide company during a treatment
- Go for a walk together or watch a movie one evening

Support Groups

For professional or personal reasons, many people with cancer may live far from their usual support network and can feel very isolated. If this describes you, don't despair; there are wonderful cancer support groups in every town and on the internet.

Support groups can:

- Take pressure off your friends, family, and caregivers by providing you with additional support
- Offer connection, information, and advice from people who have been through the same thing
- Give you the opportunity to use your knowledge to help others
- Enhance self-esteem, reduce depression, decrease anxiety, and improve relationships with family members and friends
- Help you cope better with your diagnosis and increase your knowledge of cancer and its treatment

When choosing a support group, shop around. Some groups are structured and moderated by professionals, such as psychologists, psychiatrists, oncology social workers, oncology nurses, or pastors. Others are smaller groups of people who meet informally, often led by a cancer survivor.

Once you find a group that sounds good, attend a few meetings to see how you like it. Remember that support groups can change over time as participants come and go, so even if you find one you like, evaluate it periodically to make sure it continues to meet your needs.

"Red flags" that may signal a problem with a support group include:

- Meetings that are predominantly gripe sessions
- Promises of a cure for your disease or condition
- A group leader or member who urges you to stop medical treatment
- High fees to attend the group
- Pressure to purchase products or services
- Disruptive members
- Criticism of your decisions or actions

Internet support groups have grown in popularity—particularly among young adults with cancer—thanks to accessibility, a wide audience, less commitment, and less awkwardness. An online support group may be a good choice, as long as you are discerning. Be aware that people may not be who they say they are, or may be trying to market a product or treatment. Be very careful about revealing personal information, and understand the terms of use for any site. And don't let internet use replace your in-person social network.

Online support has its limitations too, such as:

- Questionable quality: crowdsourcing medical questions may be easy and tempting, but in unmoderated forums, it's impossible to know how reliable and valid the answers are. Don't take medical advice from someone who's not a part of your medical care team.
- Frustrations about online communication: unanswered posts, unexplained disappearances, lack of nonverbal cues leading to misunderstandings, inadequate support.
- Less fulfilling connections: as much as the physical distance makes online communication less awkward and intimidating, it can also make online interaction less satisfying and meaningful than a touch or smile.
- Restricted range of conversation: online support groups may, by default, restrict the topic of conversation to cancer, rather than a more balanced variety of topics.

- Selection bias: the most vocal members might be the ones who are struggling the most. This selection bias might skew the content and tone of postings on groups.

To find a support group, check these options:

- The American Cancer Society (ACS) runs cancer support groups nationwide. You can also contact the ACS toll-free: 800-ACS-FREE (227-3733). Cancer information specialists are available 24 hours a day: cancer.org/treatment/support-programs-and-services
- ACS's Cancer Survivors Network is an online community created by and for cancer survivors and their loved ones: csn.cancer.org
- CancerCare offers professionally facilitated support groups online, over the phone, and at locations in New York (New York City & Long Island), New Jersey, and Connecticut: cancercare.org
- The National Cancer Institute offers a database of organizations that offer cancer-related services: supportorgs.cancer.gov
- The Cancer Support Community offers online support groups for patients, caregivers, and those who have completed their cancer treatment: cancersupportcommunity.org

Over to You: Connection Action Plan

- Tell family, friends, and loved ones about the type of support you need from them. Be specific; it will help them help you better.
- If you live alone, tell relatives and friends who live far away but want to support you what you would find helpful (for instance, delivery meals ordered for you from local restaurants, paying for a massage, taxi rides, or other amenities that will make your life a little easier).

- Join a support group (or several), either in person or online. Your cancer center probably offers support groups; those would be a good place to start.
- Don't feel guilty about asking for and accepting support; someday you'll be able to pay it forward.

Access Spirituality

Cancer often provokes a spiritual crisis. People may feel overwhelmed by anxiety, anger, grief, loss, and hopelessness. They must struggle with their own mortality as they face the very real questions "Will I survive?" and "What happens next?" A cancer diagnosis may shake a person's entire belief system. They may experience anger toward their God and a crisis of faith.

As cancer patients search to find meaning in lives and relationships, spirituality can help. Speaking with a religious or spiritual leader or a hospital chaplain can provide space for safe expression of anger, doubt, and fear.

Spirituality and Religion

Spirituality is the awareness of something greater than oneself. Being in touch with your spiritual self means embracing your connectedness to that which gives your life meaning and purpose.

Religion is a specific set of beliefs or practices connected to an organized group. Some people express their spirituality through organized religion. For others, spirituality involves exploring and deepening their relationship with themselves and a higher power.

Studies indicate that most patients rely upon spirituality to help them cope with their cancer and treatment. Benefits of spirituality in cancer care include:

- Decreased anxiety, depression, anger, and discomfort
- Decreased feelings of isolation, loneliness, and risk of suicide

- Increased ability to adjust to the physical and emotional effects of cancer treatments
- Increased ability to enjoy life during cancer treatment
- Increased positive feelings, including optimism, freedom from regret, satisfaction with life, and inner peace

These spiritual practices may help you cope with your cancer and its treatments:

- Taking regular time to meditate or pray, either alone or with your clergy or counselor, a meditation group, or prayer or support group
- Reading spiritual writings: the Bible, Koran, Bhagavad Gita, other faith-based texts, contemporary books on spirituality
- Listening to music that uplifts you
- Spending time in nature
- Keeping a journal

Developing a spiritual life can take a while, especially if it's new to you. Give it time. Experiment. Allow it to wax and wane. Notice how you feel when you spend time in the presence of people you love, in nature, or enjoying art or music. All these things and more can nurture your spirit and help you feel connected to yourself and the world around you.

Over to You: Spirituality Action Plan

- If you already have a spiritual practice, consider taking this opportunity to deepen it
- If you don't, talk with your friends about their spiritual life; revisit your childhood spiritual community (provided this was a place of comfort)
- Retreat to spiritual places, natural settings, art or nature museums, or any place that helps you cultivate a sense of peace
- Keep a journal where you can reflect on the journey you're on

- Read books by Bernie Siegel, M.D., a retired surgeon who has written several inspirational books about the relationship between the patient and the healing process, including *Love, Medicine and Miracles* and *Faith, Hope and Healing*

Chapter 10

Beyond Treatment

The last day of your cancer treatment isn't the end of your cancer journey. Even though you may want to never think about cancer again, a survivorship care plan will help you transition into the post-treatment phase of your healing journey.

Follow-up Care Plan

Your oncology team will provide you with a summary of your treatments received and a follow-up care plan that summarizes potential late effects, recommendations for future cancer screening, and more.

When you receive your follow-up care plan, the National Cancer Institute recommends that you ask any other questions you may have, such as:

- How long will it take for me to get better and feel more like myself?
- Which doctor(s) should I see for my follow-up care? How often?
- What symptoms should I watch out for?
- What tests do I need after treatment is over? How often will I have them?
- What are long-term health issues I might expect as a result of my cancer treatment?
- What is the chance that my cancer will return?

- What records do I need to keep about my treatment?
- What can I do to take care of myself and be as healthy as possible?
- Can you suggest a support group that might help me?

Take notes or record your talks for later referral. Talk about any concerns you have related to your follow-up care plan.

Between scheduled visits, be aware of any changes in your health. Report any problems to your doctor immediately. During follow-up visits, talk openly about:

- Any physical problems that interfere with your daily life, such as fatigue; problems with bladder, bowel, or sexual function; having a hard time concentrating; memory changes; trouble sleeping; weight gain or loss
- Any new medicines, vitamins, herbs, or supplements you're taking
- Changes in your family medical history
- Any emotional problems, such as anxiety or depression

Keep in mind, however, that new symptoms don't necessarily mean the cancer has come back. Your doctor can determine whether the problems are related to the cancer, the treatment you received, or an unrelated health issue.

Functional Medicine to Improve Your Odds

Unfortunately, people who have or had cancer have a higher risk of dying from any cause than people who have never had cancer. If that worries you, take heart: You can significantly reduce that risk with functional medicine.

Functional medicine is the use of lab tests, lifestyle habits, and other interventions, including drugs, nutritional and other complementary therapies, and technology, to identify your personal health profile and create a targeted plan to improve your health and reduce cancer risk.

Functional medicine tests and techniques, sometimes called "biohacking," may include:

- Health risk assessment, including hereditary, epigenetic age, and cardiovascular risks
- Micronutrient assessment
- Hormonal analysis
- Gut microbiome evaluation
- Sensitive diagnostic and screening technologies to look for cancer in its earliest stages
- Wearable devices to evaluate physical activity, body measurements, sleep quality, and more (see Resources: Apps and Devices, p. 273)
- Drug sensitivity testing

Data from these methods can guide your use of different evidence-based interventions. For example, functional medicine information may help:

- Improve the anticancer effectiveness of immunotherapies
- Target cancer-cell metabolism with specific off-label drugs (see p. 17) and supplements
- Reduce your risk of cancer metastases from cancer surgery or biopsy

If you choose to use Dr. Lawenda's Integrative Oncology Essentials program, some lab tests can be shipped directly to your home, or we can coordinate lab testing at sites close to you. You can also sign up for a phone or video consultation to interpret your lab results and improve your cancer outcome or general health. Find out more at **ioeprogram.com/lab-tests**.

Diet and Lifestyle Changes for Life

Once your treatment ends, we encourage you to shift to a lifestyle that reduces the risks of cancer coming back, comprising:

- A nutrient-dense diet
- Daily exercise
- Restful sleep
- Optimal circadian rhythms
- Tools to manage stress

- A reduced toxic load, and
- Close connection with others

As we state throughout the book, it takes time to change old habits, so don't pressure yourself to adopt several new habits overnight. Start with easy changes and progress gradually.

At any point along the way, you might find it helpful to work with a coach, therapist, or medical expert to help you stay on track. Dr. Lawenda and Conner offer online programs for people who have finished cancer treatment and want to reduce their risk of recurrence; check our websites to find out more, and sign up to our mailing lists to be alerted of forthcoming courses.

Alternatively, ask a friend—perhaps someone who's on a similar journey with cancer—to be your health buddy; you can trade recipes and cook meals together, exercise together, attend courses together and provide each other with a combination of support and accountability.

End-of-Life Preparations

Despite major treatment advances, many people eventually die from cancer. Having end-of-life conversations is emotional for all involved, but it's important and empowering to address these important questions when you're not rushed or in an emergency situation.

Advance Directives

Every adult should have an advance directive that explains the type of healthcare you do or do not want when you're unable to communicate your wishes. Advance directives could include:

A living will. This alerts medical professionals and your family to the treatments you want to receive or refuse (such as artificial life support, feeding tubes, and kidney dialysis). In most states this document only goes into effect if you meet specific medical criteria and are unable to make decisions.

A healthcare power of attorney or healthcare proxy. You select a family member or trusted friend to make healthcare decisions for you when you cannot. In this document you give directions to the person you select about your healthcare wishes. (Download forms here: aarp.org/caregiving/financial-legal/free-printable-advance-directives/)

After-death details, such as funeral arrangements, burial services, notifications to family and friends, special messages, and memorials.

Financial affairs, including wills, documents, insurance policies, bank accounts, investment summaries, car and house titles, passwords to online accounts (and what to do with those accounts).

End-of-life plans and discussions can also include:

- Counseling support or spiritual guidance, as part of hospice care or at bedside on occasion
- Desired accomplishments before you pass, such as travel or enjoying certain experiences; these can help bring a sense of meaning and completion
- People you wish to see or talk to; this can bring an important sense of comfort, meaning, completion, and peace

Hospice and Palliative Care

Hospice is an important service (fully paid for by Medicare and many private insurance plans) for anyone with six months or less to live. Hospice provides support (not curative treatments) for pain and other symptoms, emotional and psychological issues, and spiritual needs. Hospice teams often include doctors, nurses, social workers, nutritionists, and chaplains. Care can be delivered in a hospice facility, hospital, nursing home, or someone's home.

Palliative care can be provided alongside curative treatments and may begin at any time in the course of a disease. When palliative care is no longer helping, the person can transition to hospice care or continue to receive palliative care with an increased emphasis on comfort care.

Death with Dignity

Death with dignity laws, also known as physician-assisted dying or aid-in-dying laws, enable terminally ill people to determine how much pain and suffering they want to endure. Death with dignity statutes allow mentally competent adults with a confirmed prognosis of six or fewer months to live to voluntarily request and receive a prescription medication to hasten their inevitable, imminent death. The protections in the statutes ensure that patients remain the driving force in end-of-life care discussions.

As of early 2021, California, Colorado, District of Columbia, Hawaii, Maine, New Jersey, Oregon, Vermont, and Washington have physician-assisted dying statutes. Learn more about the death with dignity programs from the Death with Dignity National Center (deathwithdignity.org/faqs/).

Chapter 11

Resources

We have mentioned resources and useful web links throughout this book; here is a list—by no means complete—of the ones we consider particularly important or useful.

Our Websites

- The IOE (Integrative Oncology Essentials) Online Program (ioeprogram.com) is Dr. Lawenda's educational course covering many of the topics in this handbook and much more. You will learn everything you need to empower your cancer journey and improve your overall health. Additionally, video and phone consultations with Dr. Lawenda, as well as functional medicine lab testing, are available.
- Dr. Lawenda's website, with wide-ranging articles about cancer and its treatments: integrativeoncology-essentials.com.
- Conner's website, providing articles, recipes, and nutrition coaching services for individuals and groups: modernmediterranean.com.

Apps and Devices

Exercise

- 7-Minute Workout: 7minuteworkout.jnj.com
- Miranda Esmonde-White's "Aging Backwards" workouts: on essentrics.com

Nutrition

- Cronometer: cronometer.com
- Dexcom Continuous Glucose Monitor: dexcom.com
- FreeStyle Libre Continuous Glucose Monitor: freestylelibre.us
- NIH Body Weight Planner: niddk.nih.gov/bwp
- Optimising Nutrition Macro Calculator: optimisingnutrition.com/macro-calculator

Sleep

- CBT for Insomnia: cbtforinsomnia.com
- Chilipad Ooler Blanket: chilitechnology.com
- Cleveland Clinic GoToSleep: clevelandclinicwellness.com/gotosleep
- Oura Ring: ouraring.com
- Sleepio: sleepio.com

Stress relief

- Meditation app: Calm.com
- Sleep tracker and meditation aid Muse: choosemuse.com
- Ten Percent Happier: tenpercent.com
- Waking Up: wakingup.com

Books

- *After Cancer Care* by Gerald Lemole, M.D., Pallav Mehta, M.D., and Dwight McKee, M.D.
- *Always Hungry?* by Dr. David Ludwig and Dawn Ludwig
- *Anticancer: A New Way of Life* by David Servan-Schreiber, M.D., PhD (see also the 2015 documentary *The C-Word*, about David Servan-Schreiber's life and work)
- *Anticancer Living* by Lorenzo Cohen, M.D., and Alison Jefferies, M.Ed.
- *Autoimmune Wellness Handbook* by Mickey Trescott and Angie Alt
- *Body by Science* by John Little and Doug McGuff, M.D.
- *Eat to Beat Disease: The New Science of How Your Body Can Heal Itself* by William Li, M.D.
- *Integrative Oncology* by Donald Abrams, M.D.
- *Keto for Cancer* by Miriam Kalamian
- *Life Over Cancer* by Keith Block, M.D.
- *The Definitive Guide to Cancer* and *The Definitive Guide to Thriving After Cancer* by Lise Alschuler, N.D., and Karolyn Gazella
- *The Obesity Code* and *The Cancer Code* by Jason Fung, M.D.
- *The Metabolic Approach to Cancer* by Nasha Winters, N.D., and Jess Higgins Kelley, MNT
- *Zest for Life: The Mediterranean Anticancer Diet* by Conner Middelmann-Whitney

Other Websites

By topic, listed alphabetically

Aspirin

- *Regular Aspirin Use May Increase Older People's Risk of Dying from Cancer* (U.S. National Cancer Institute, https://www.cancer.gov/news-events/cancer-currents-blog/2020/aspree-aspirin-increases-advanced-cancer#:~:text=This%20widespread%20use%20of%20aspirin,prevention%20potential%2C%20including%20for%20cancer.)
- *Daily aspirin therapy: Understand the benefits and risks* (Mayo Clinic, http://www.mayoclinic.com/health/daily-aspirin-therapy/HB00073)
- *Aspirin* (U.S. National Institutes of Health, http://www.nlm.nih.gov/medlineplus/druginfo/meds/a682878.html)
- *The Everyday Drug That Prevents Cancer Death* (Life Extension article, 2011, https://www.lifeextension.com/magazine/2011/5/the-everyday-drug-that-prevents-cancer-death)

Breast Health

- American Society of Breast Surgeons Consensus Guideline on Genetic Testing for Hereditary Breast Cancer (https://www.breastsurgeons.org/docs/statements/Consensus-Guideline-on-Genetic-Testing-for-Hereditary-Breast-Cancer.pdf)
- *BRCA Analysis* (Myriad Genetics–Patient Information, http://www.bracnow.com)
- *BRCA1 and BRCA2: Cancer Risk and Genetic Testing* (U.S. National Cancer Institute, http://www.cancer.gov/cancertopics/factsheet/Risk/BRCA)

- *BRCA Screening* (Susan G. Komen Foundation–Patient Information, http://ww5.komen.org/BreastCancer/GeneMutationsampGeneticTesting.html)
- *Breastcancer.org* (Information on preventive mastectomy, http://www.breastcancer.org/treatment/surgery/prophylactic_mast.jsp)
- *Breastfree.org*: A nonprofit website for women who want to learn more about living breast-free. Here, you'll find the information you need to select breast forms, bras, and swimsuits. You'll find advice about creative ways to look good and feel great about yourself. And you'll find support from women who have chosen not to reconstruct and want to share their stories with you (http://breastfree.org/index.php).
- *Foodforbreastcancer.com*: A nonprofit website providing information on how various foods and other factors affect breast cancer risk, prevention, and prognosis. Findings are drawn exclusively from scientific studies and updated as new research becomes available. Includes in-depth articles on what to eat for various types of breast cancer (e.g., HER2 overexpressing, ER+/PR+, triple-negative, or lobular) and during treatment (radiation, Taxol, aromatase inhibitor). (http://www.foodforbreastcancer.com)
- *Inherited Risk for Breast & Ovarian Cancers* (Memorial Sloan Kettering Cancer Center, http://www.mskcc.org/cancer-care/hereditary-genetics/inherited-risk-breast-ovarian)
- *National Cancer Institute* (Fact sheet on preventive mastectomy, http://www.cancer.gov/cancertopics/factsheet/Therapy/preventive-mastectomy)
- *Susan G. Komen* (Information on preventive mastectomy, http://ww5.komen.org/BreastCancer/PreventiveSurgery.html)

Cancer Distress Support Resources:

- *American Psychosocial Oncology Society*: A place where patients and caregivers can obtain referrals to psychological resources in their community (https://apos-society.org/)
- *CancerCare.org*: Professional oncology social workers provide support, information, and resources to help you better cope with cancer (https://www.cancercare.org/)
- *American Association of Marriage and Family Therapy*. This organization has a searchable database that lists marriage and family therapists in the United States and abroad (https://www.aamft.org/)
- *Association of Oncology Social Work*. This organization provides a list of qualified oncology social workers in your area (https://aosw.org/)
- *American Psychological Association*. This organization offers an online psychologist locator service (https://www.apa.org/)
- *Mental Health America*. This organization provides a directory of local mental health associations that connect clients with mental health services (https://www.mhanational.org/)
- *National Register of Health Service Providers in Psychology*. This organization's searchable database (findapsychologist.org) helps people locate doctoral-level psychologists in the United States and Canada

Cannabis

- Here's a great article on the development of Sativex. (http://motherjones.com/politics/2005/11/respectable-reefer)
- Article on the differences between Marinol (synthetic marijuana) and cannabis (http://norml.org/marijuana/medical/marinol-vs-natural-cannabis); **Summary of key points**: 1) Marinol lacks several of the therapeutic

compounds available in cannabis; 2) Marinol is more psychoactive than cannabis; 3) Cannabis vaporization offers advantages over orally administered THC; 4) Marinol is more expensive than cannabis; and 5) Patients prefer cannabis to Marinol.

- Excellent documentary: *What if Cannabis Cured Cancer?* (http://www.amazon.com/What-If-Cannabis-Cured-Cancer/dp/B003SSBSQQ/ref=atv_dvd_twister) Dr. Andrew Weil (http://www.integrativeoncology-essentials.com/2012/01/cannabis-and-cancer-1-plant-versus-5-common-symptoms-that-affect-cancer-patients/) summarizes the remarkable research findings of recent years about the cancer-protective effects of novel compounds in marijuana. Most medical doctors are not aware of this information and its implications for prevention and treatment. This documentary presents compelling evidence that our current policy on cannabis is counterproductive and foolish. An excellent film." Available to stream on Amazon. (50 minutes; 2011).
- MontanaPBS's documentary, *Clearing the Smoke: The Science of Cannabis*, reveals how cannabis acts on the brain and in the body to treat nausea, pain, epilepsy, and potentially even cancer. Extensive interviews with patients, doctors, researchers, and skeptics detail the promises and the limitations of medicinal cannabis. (57 minutes. February 2011, http://watch.montanapbs.org/video/1825223761)

Chemotherapy-Induced Peripheral Neuropathy (CIPN):

- *Neuropathy Care For Cancer Survivors* (Memorial Sloan Kettering Cancer Center http://www.mskcc.org/videos/playlist/neuropathy-care-survivors): Great four-part video on helping survivors better understand the treatment and management of neuropathy

- *Chemotherapy Neuropathy Treatment* (Beating Neuropathy Radio http://www.blogtalkradio.com/bnradio/2013/03/10/chemotherapy-neuropathy-treatment)
- *Managing Peripheral Neuropathy* (Cancer.net/all-about-cancer/cancernet-feature-articles/side-effects/managing-peripheral-neuropathy)
- *Chemotherapy-Induced Neuropathy* (NCI Cancer Bulletin https://www.cancer.gov/about-cancer/treatment/side-effects/nerve-problems)
- *Peripheral Neuropathy Caused By Chemotherapy* (American Cancer Society http://www.cancer.org/treatment/treatmentsandsideeffects/physicalsideeffects/chemotherapyeffects/peripheralneuropathy/peripheral-neuropathy-caused-by-chemotherapy-toc)

Cold Cap Therapy

- *The Rapunzel Project* (http://www.rapunzelproject.org/Default.aspx) is a wonderful nonprofit organization that was established to help chemotherapy patients maintain their hair during treatment. They have also helped to get funding for CCT freezers. Check out their useful tips (http://www.rapunzelproject.org/ColdCaps.aspx#HelpfulTips) for CCT users and their list of cancer centers that have cold cap freezers: rapunzelproject.org/ColdCaps/Locations.aspx.
- *BreastCancer.org Community Posts* (http://community.breastcancer.org/posts/search; type in "cold caps" in the search tab and you will find thousands of posts discussing cold caps)
- *Penguin Cold Cap Therapy* (https://penguincoldcaps.com/)
- *DigniCap CCT system* (http://www.dignitana.com/)
- *ChemoCap* (http://www.chemocap.com/)
- *Elasto-Gel Cold Caps* (https://www.elastogels.com/)
- *Paxman (PCS-1 and 2, Orbis)* (http://www.paxman-coolers.co.uk/)

- *Chemocoldcaps* (a full-service U.S.-based company that sells a package that includes delivery of Elasto-Gel cold caps, all the supplies and accessories you'll need, and personalized training and tips to provide you the best outcome possible, http://www.chemocoldcaps.com/)

Herbal Medicines Berberine & Goldenseal

- *Examine.com* (berberine, http://examine.com/supplements/Berberine)
- *Healthline* (goldenseal, https://www.healthline.com/health/goldenseal-cure-for-everything)
- *Healthline* (berberine, https://www.healthline.com/nutrition/berberine-powerful-supplement)
- *Memorial Sloan Kettering Cancer Center: About Herbs* (goldenseal, http://www.mskcc.org/cancer-care/herb/goldenseal)
- *"Clinical Applications for Berberine: Potential therapeutic applications in metabolic syndrome, type 2 diabetes, and dyslipidemia," Natural Medicine Journal*, December 2012 (Jacob Schor, ND FABNO, https://www.naturalmedicinejournal.com/journal/2012-12/clinical-applications-berberine)

International Resources

- *International Agency for Research on Cancer (http://www.iarc.fr)*

Melatonin in Cancer Care

- *U.S. National Institutes of Health* (http://www.clinicaltrials.gov/ct2/results?term=melatonin+and+cancer&Search=Search)
- *Memorial Sloan Kettering Cancer Center (About Herbs)* (http://www.mskcc.org/cancer-care/herb/melatonin)
- *Melatonin, Chronobiology and Cancer* (a presentation by Drs. Hrushesky, Blask, and Lissoni, https://cam.cancer.gov/docs/MelatoninSummary-508.pdf)

- *"Melatonin and Cancer Treatment"* (Life Extension article, 2004, https://www.lifeextension.com/magazine/2004/1/report_melatonin)

Nutrition & Diet

- Optimising Nutrition Cancer recipe books: (app.optimisingnutrition.com/cancer-recipe-books) Quick and easy meals designed specifically for cancer patients and survivors. Dr. Lawenda collaborated with nutrition expert Marty Kendall (optimsingnutrition.com) on three recipe books which focus on nutrient density.
- American Cancer Society Guidelines for Diet and Physical Activity: *American Institute for Cancer Research* (https://www.aicr.org/cancer-prevention/)

Resources in Canada

- *Health Canada Hotlist* (http://environmentaldefence.ca/issues/just-beautiful/glossary)
- *David Suzuki Foundation Dirty Dozen* (http://www.davidsuzuki.org/issues/health/science/toxics/dirty-dozen-cosmetic-chemicals)
- *Canadian Centre for Occupational Health & Safety* (http://ccinfoweb.ccohs.ca/chemindex/search.html)
- *Environment Canada Domestic Substance List* (http://www.ec.gc.ca/lcpe-cepa/default.asp?lang=En&n=0DA2924D-1)

Sleep

- *"How to Sleep Better: Tips for Getting a Good Night's Sleep"* (great summary of tips for better sleep, https://www.helpguide.org/articles/sleep/getting-better-sleep.htm)

- *"How Foods Affect Our Sleep"* (The New York Times, December 2020, https://www.nytimes.com/2020/12/10/well/eat/sleep-foods-diet.html)
- *"11 Exercises for Better Sleep"* (The New York Times, October 2020, https://www.nytimes.com/2020/10/10/at-home/exercises-for-better-sleep.html)
- *"How a Lack of Sleep May Increase Calorie Consumption"* (Sleep Foundation, December 2020, https://www.sleepfoundation.org/sleep-deprivation/lack-sleep-may-increase-calorie-consumption)

Spirituality and Cancer

- *Spirituality in Cancer Care* (National Cancer Institute PDQ)
- *Finding Meaning* (https://www.dana-farber.org/for-patients-and-families/for-survivors/caring-for-yourself-after-cancer/finding-meaning) and *Spiritual Care* (https://www.dana-farber.org/for-patients-and-families/care-and-treatment/support-services-and-amenities/spiritual-care/) (Dana-Farber Cancer Institute)
- Finding Comfort in Spirituality (National Comprehensive Cancer Network, https://www.nccn.org/patients/resources/life_with_cancer/spirituality.aspx#:~:text=Experts%20say%20that%20spiritual%20or,and%20feelings%20of%20inner%20peace.)
- *"FICA" Spiritual Assessment Tool* developed to help physicians and other healthcare professionals address spiritual issues with patients. They also have a great online course, *Spiritual Assessment in Clinical Practice*, for healthcare providers on learning about how to do a spiritual assessment: assessing the spiritual beliefs, values, and practices important in your patients' responses to illness or stress. (The George Washington Institute for Spirituality and Health, https://smhs.gwu.edu/spirituality-health/program/transforming-practice-health-settings/clinical-fica-tool)

Stress Reduction References

- *Anxiety* (Oncology Nursing Society, http://www.ons.org/Research/PEP/Anxiety)
- *Caregiver Strain/Burden* (Oncology Nursing Society, https://www.ons.org/pep/caregiver-strain-and-burden)
- *Coping with Emotional and Physical Concerns* (a great reference by Cancer.Net, http://www.cancer.net/patient/Coping/Emotional+and+Physical+Matters)
- *"Integrative Oncology: Complementary Therapies for Pain, Anxiety, and Mood Disturbance"* by Gary Deng, Barrie R Cassileth (https://pubmed.ncbi.nlm.nih.gov/15761079/#:~:text=Complementary%20therapies%20such%20as%20acupuncture,to%20relieve%20chronic%20cancer%20pain)
- *"Stress, Depression, The Immune System and Cancer,"* excellent overview by Edna Maria Vissoci Reiche et al. (https://www.thelancet.com/journals/lanonc/article/PIIS1470-2045(04)01597-9/fulltext)
- *Psychological stress and cancer* (National Cancer Institute fact sheet , http://www.cancer.gov/cancertopics/factsheet/Risk/stress)
- *"The Value of Acupuncture in Cancer Care"* by Weidong Lu et al. (https://www.ncbi.nlm.nih.gov/pmc/articles/PMC2642987/?tool=pubmed)
- *Acupuncture significantly reduces anxiety* with a simple 5-minute treatment (http://www.integrativeoncology-essentials.com/anxiety-stress-can-be-reduced-with-a-simple-5-minute-acupuncture-treatment)
- *Anxiety, Fear and Depression* (American Cancer Society, http://www.cancer.org/docroot/MBC/MBC_4x_Anxiety.asp)
- *Post-Traumatic Stress Disorder and Cancer* (https://www.cancer.net/survivorship/life-after-cancer/post-traumatic-stress-disorder-and-cancer)
- *Taking Care of Yourself Under Stress* (University of Minnesota Extension, https://extension.umn.edu/taking-care-yourself-under-stress)

Toxins

- Beauty without Bunnies: Animal-derived ingredients, PETA (http://www.peta.org/living/beauty-and-personal-care/companies/2657.aspx)
- *Beyond Pesticides*: Information on pesticides and alternatives to their use (http://www.beyondpesticides.org)
- *Campaign for Safe Cosmetics* (http://www.safecosmetics.org)
- *Cancer Council Australia* on pesticides and cancer (http://wiki.cancer.org.au/prevention/Position_statement_-_Pesticides_and_cancer)
- *CHE Toxicant and Disease Database* (http://www.healthandenvironment.org/tddb)
- *Cosmetic Ingredient Review Assessment* (http://www.cir-safety.org)
- *National Cancer Institute* (https://www.cancer.gov/about-cancer/causes-prevention/risk/substances)
- *National Toxicology Program Report on Carcinogens* (https://ntp.niehs.nih.gov/whatwestudy/assessments/cancer/roc/index.html)
- *PAN/Pesticide Action Network*: Works to replace the use of hazardous pesticides with ecologically sound and socially just alternatives (http://www.panna.org)
- *Proposition 65 The Safe Drinking Water and Toxic Enforcement Act of 1986* (http://oehha.ca.gov/prop65/law/P65law72003.html)
- *US Environmental Protection Agency* (Pesticides, http://www.epa.gov/pesticides))
- *Women's Voices for the Earth* (Toxic chemicals in day-to-day products, http://www.womensvoices.org/avoid-toxic-chemicals/15-toxic-trespassers)
- *World Health Organization* (Pesticides, http://www.who.int/topics/pesticides/en)

Index

Made in the USA
Middletown, DE
11 March 2023

26611800R00172